BIOPHYSICS
in
Nursing

BIOPHYSICS in Nursing

As per the INC Syllabus for Post Basic BSc Nursing

Second Edition

Suresh K Sharma MScN PhD FNRS RN (USA)
Professor and Principal
College of Nursing
All India Institute of Medical Sciences (AIIMS)
Jodhpur, Rajasthan, India

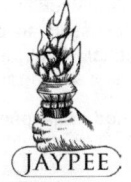

JAYPEE BROTHERS MEDICAL PUBLISHERS
The Health Sciences Publisher
New Delhi | London

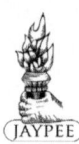 **Jaypee Brothers Medical Publishers (P) Ltd**

Headquarters
Jaypee Brothers Medical Publishers (P) Ltd
EMCA House, 23/23-B
Ansari Road, Daryaganj
New Delhi 110 002, India
Landline: +91-11-23272143, +91-11-23272703
+91-11-23282021, +91-11-23245672
Email: jaypee@jaypeebrothers.com

Corporate Office
Jaypee Brothers Medical Publishers (P) Ltd
4838/24, Ansari Road, Daryaganj
New Delhi 110 002, India
Phone: +91-11-43574357
Fax: +91-11-43574314
Email: jaypee@jaypeebrothers.com

Overseas Office
J.P. Medical Ltd
83 Victoria Street, London
SW1H 0HW (UK)
Phone: +44 20 3170 8910
Fax: +44 (0)20 3008 6180
Email: info@jpmedpub.com

Website: www.jaypeebrothers.com
Website: www.jaypeedigital.com

© 2023, Jaypee Brothers Medical Publishers

The views and opinions expressed in this book are solely those of the original contributor(s)/author(s) and do not necessarily represent those of editor(s) and publisher of the book.

All rights reserved. No part of this publication may be reproduced, stored or transmitted in any form or by any means, electronic, mechanical, photocopying, recording or otherwise, without the prior permission in writing of the publishers.

All brand names and product names used in this book are trade names, service marks, trademarks or registered trademarks of their respective owners. The publisher is not associated with any product or vendor mentioned in this book.

Medical knowledge and practice change constantly. This book is designed to provide accurate, authoritative information about the subject matter in question. However, readers are advised to check the most current information available on procedures included and check information from the manufacturer of each product to be administered, to verify the recommended dose, formula, method and duration of administration, adverse effects and contraindications. It is the responsibility of the practitioner to take all appropriate safety precautions. Neither the publisher nor the author(s)/editor(s) assume any liability for any injury and/or damage to persons or property arising from or related to use of material in this book.

This book is sold on the understanding that the publisher is not engaged in providing professional medical services. If such advice or services are required, the services of a competent medical professional should be sought.

Every effort has been made where necessary to contact holders of copyright to obtain permission to reproduce copyright material. If any have been inadvertently overlooked, the publisher will be pleased to make the necessary arrangements at the first opportunity.

Inquiries for bulk sales may be solicited at: jaypee@jaypeebrothers.com

Biophysics in Nursing
First Edition: **2011**
Second Edition: **2023**
ISBN: 978-93-5696-102-9

Printed at: Sterling Graphics Pvt. Ltd. India

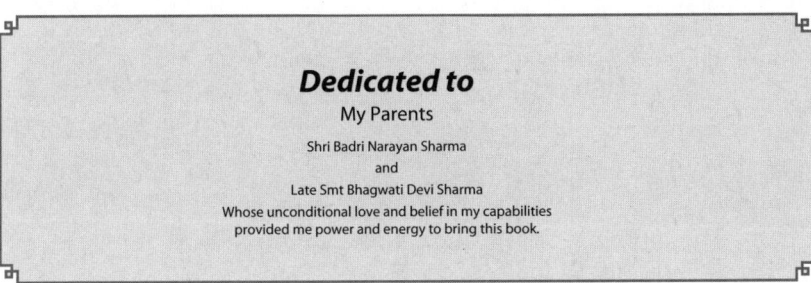

Dedicated to
My Parents

Shri Badri Narayan Sharma
and
Late Smt Bhagwati Devi Sharma

Whose unconditional love and belief in my capabilities
provided me power and energy to bring this book.

Contributors

Mrs Navjot Kaur MScN
Assistant Professor
College of Nursing
All India Institute of Medical Sciences
Deoghar, Jharkhand, India

Dr Shiv Kumar Mudgal PhD
Associate Professor
College of Nursing
All India Institute of Medical Sciences
Deoghar, Jharkhand, India

Dr Rakhi Gaur PhD
Assistant Professor
College of Nursing
All India Institute of Medical Sciences
Deoghar, Jharkhand, India

Reviewers

Er Kishor Kumar Sharma M Tech
Ex-Fellow, Indian Institute of Technology (IIT)
Kharagpur, West Bengal, India

Ms Monika Stephen BScN
Nursing Tutor
College of Nursing
Dayanand Medical College and Hospital
Ludhiana, Punjab, India

Er Kuldeep Gautam B Tech
Ex-Fellow, KIIT University
Bhubaneswar, Odisha, India

Er Prashant S Geel B Tech
Malaviya National Institute of Technology
Jaipur, Rajasthan, India

Dr Satyaveer Rulania PhD
Tutor
College of Nursing
All India Institute of Medical Sciences
Jodhpur, Rajasthan, India

Preface to the Second Edition

Biophysics is a growing enterprise worldwide, driven primarily by the widespread realization of the major contribution that can be made to biological science by a combination of truly state-of-the-art physical measurements. The field occupies a unique and central position at the intersection of the physical, and medical sciences.

Indian nursing students and educators rely heavily on books written by the medical and engineering fraternity, especially in the fields of biophysics. This is because the books written by these groups have a lot of high-quality content. Due to differences in their curricula, the content published by the medical and engineering fraternities is only partially applicable to the Indian nursing fraternity. As a result, an idea was conceived to create a book on Biophysics that is rich in quality and excellence, at par with international standards, and suitable for Indian nursing students and educators.

After writing few books, it might have grown tedious for me to rewrite material that has been written a million times by numerous accomplished authors. However, the process of rewriting this amazing and priceless book for the nursing community turned out to be a great learning opportunity.

This revised edition titled *Biophysics in Nursing* is a modest attempt to reorganize the sequence and content of chapters as per the syllabi designed by Indian Nursing Council for Post Basic BSc Nursing. The chapters are enriched with basic principles and practices of biophysics in simple, lucid and illustrative manner by incorporating their applications to healthcare and nursing practices.

The content in textbook included chapters on basic physical principles and healthcare/nursing applications of biophysics, motions, gravity, force, energy, work, heat, light, pressure, sound, electricity, electromagnetism, atomic energy and electronics.

I believe the updated edition of this book will be able to meet the requirements of Indian nursing students and educators while also giving readers useful content planning for various competitive exams for jobs or higher education.

Suresh K Sharma

Preface to the First Edition

Biophysics is a growing enterprise worldwide, driven primarily by the widespread realization of the major contribution that can be made to biological science by a combination of truly state-of-the-art physical measurements with modern molecular biology. The field occupies a unique and central position at the intersection of the biological, chemical, physical, and medical sciences.

Most of human biological functions or healthcare practices have the basis of principles of biophysics. Therefore, nurses involved in providing nursing care must understand the physical principles and their applications in healthcare practices. So that, nurses can assess, plan, implement and evaluate each care intervention more effectively and scientifically.

This textbook titled *Biophysics in Nursing* is a modest attempt to bring about the basic physical principles in a simple, non-mathematical approach by incorporating their applications to healthcare and nursing practices. It has been ensured that each physical principle is simply defined and discussed with its application to nursing practices. Each topic of the content is presented in a simple and lucid manner by using illustrations and examples from healthcare and nursing practice areas. The content of this textbook will fully meet the needs of the nursing students studying in the Post Basic BSc Nursing program since it is designed on the revised syllabus of the Indian Nursing Council, New Delhi. In addition, it will be also useful for the nurses planning for different competitive exams for jobs or higher studies.

Suresh K Sharma

Contents

Chapter 1: Introduction to Biophysics   1
Suresh K Sharma, Navjot Kaur
- ❖ Meaning of Biophysics 2
- ❖ Importance of Biophysics in Nursing 2
- ❖ Concept of Units 5
- ❖ Fundamental and Derived Units 5
- ❖ Systems of Units 6
- ❖ Fundamental Units in Various Systems 6

Chapter 2: Motion   13
Suresh K Sharma, Navjot Kaur
- ❖ Scalars and Vectors 13
- ❖ Rest and Motion 15
- ❖ Speed 16
- ❖ Velocity 16
- ❖ Acceleration 17
- ❖ Applications of Motion in Nursing 18

Chapter 3: Gravity   21
Suresh K Sharma, Navjot Kaur
- ❖ Specific Gravity 22
- ❖ Center of Gravity 23
- ❖ Mass and Weight 24
- ❖ Principles of Gravity 26
- ❖ Applications of Archimedes' Principle 28
- ❖ Effects of Gravitational Forces on the Human Body and Application of Principles of Gravity in Nursing 28

Chapter 4: Force, Energy and Work   34
Suresh K Sharma, Navjot Kaur
- ❖ Force 34
- ❖ Units of Measurement 35
- ❖ Newton's Law of Motion 35
- ❖ Principles of Friction 40
- ❖ Forces in the Circular Motion 41
- ❖ Work 44
- ❖ Energy 45
- ❖ Types and Transformation of Energy 46
- ❖ Energy in the Body 47
- ❖ Conservation of Energy 48
- ❖ Power 49

- Principles of Machines 49
- Efficiency and Mechanical Advantage of a Machine 50
- Body Mechanics 50
- Lever 51
- Lever Action of Jaw 53
- Lever Action of Foot 53
- Lever Action of Forearm 54
- Pulley 57
- Traction 57
- Inclined Plane 61
- Wedge 62
- Screw 62
- Application of Principles of Gravity in Nursing 62

Chapter 5: Heat   65
Navjot Kaur, Suresh K Sharma
- Nature of Heat 65
- Measurement of Heat 66
- Transfer of Heat 68
- Effects of Heat on Matter 71
- Humidity 73
- Specific Heat 74
- Temperature Scales 75
- Regulation of Body Temperature 77
- Use of Heat for Sterilization 79
- Application of Heat Principles in Nursing 79

Chapter 6: Light   84
Suresh K Sharma, Navjot Kaur
- Nature of Light 84
- Law of Reflection and Refraction of Light 88
- Lenses 92
- The Physics of Vision 94
- Defects of Vision and Its Corrections 97
- Biological Effects of the Light 100
- Uses of Light in Therapy 104
- Ultraviolet Radiation 107
- X-rays 108
- Photosensitivity 110
- Application of Principles of Light in Nursing 110

Chapter 7: Pressure and Fluid Mechanics   113
Navjot Kaur, Shiv Kumar Mudgal
- Importance of Pressure in the Human Body 114
- Atmospheric Pressure 115
- Hydrostatic Pressure 119
- Pressure in Flowing Fluids 121

❖ Osmotic Pressure 122
❖ Measurement of Pressures 125
❖ Applications of These Pressures in Nursing 130

Chapter 8: Sound Waves 132
Rakhi Gaur, Navjot Kaur
❖ Mechanism of Propagation of Waves 133
❖ Types of Waves 134
❖ Types of Wave Motion 134
❖ Sound Waves 137
❖ Some Important Terms Connected with Wave Motion 138
❖ Wave Phenomenon 140
❖ Characteristics of Sound 142
❖ Vocalization and Hearing 144
❖ Doppler Effect 145
❖ Applications 146
❖ Noise Pollution and Its Prevention 152

Chapter 9: Electricity and Electromagnetism 158
Suresh K Sharma, Navjot Kaur
❖ Types of Electricity 159
❖ Sources of Electric Current 168
❖ Effects of Electric Current 171
❖ Effects of Electricity on the Human Body 173
❖ Magnetism 174
❖ Applications of the Magnet and Magnetism 178
❖ Electroencephalography 179
❖ Electrocardiography 181
❖ Phonocardiography 182
❖ Electromyography 183
❖ Electromyography Pattern 183
❖ Electrostimulation 184
❖ Electroconvulsive Therapy 184
❖ Electronic Cardiac Pacemaker 185
❖ Brain Pacemaker 186
❖ Defibrillation 187
❖ Automated External Defibrillator 189
❖ Magnetic Resonance Imaging 191
❖ Cat Scan 193

Chapter 10: Nuclear Physics 197
Suresh K Sharma, Navjot Kaur
❖ Structure of Atom 197
❖ Radiation and Radioisotopes 206
❖ Radiation Protection Limits 218
❖ Instruments used for Detection of Ionizing Radiation, X-rays 221

Chapter 11: Electronics in Nursing   **224**
Suresh K Sharma, Rakhi Gaur
- Principles of Electronics   *225*
- Capacitors   *227*
- Transistors   *229*
- Transducers   *230*
- Common Electric Equipment Used in Patient Care   *231*

Index   *239*

INC Syllabus
Biophysics

Placement: First Year Post Basic BSc Nursing

Time Allotted:
Section A (Biochemistry): Theory 30 Hours
Section B (Biophysics): Theory 30 Hours

Biophysics

Theory: 30 hours

COURSE CONTENTS

Chapter 1
- **Introduction:** Concepts of unit and measurements
- Fundamental and derived units
- Units of length, weight, mass, time

Chapter 2
- Vector and scalar motion, speed, velocity and acceleration

Chapter 3
- **Gravity:** Specific gravity, center of gravity, principles of gravity
- Effect of gravitational forces on human body
- Application of principles of gravity in nursing

Chapter 4
- **Force, Work, Energy:** Their units of measurement
- Type and transformation of energy, forces of the body, static forces
- Principles of machines, friction and body mechanics
- Simple mechanics-lever and body mechanics, pulley and traction, incline plane, screw
- Application of these principles in nursing

Chapter 5

- **Heat:** Nature, measurement, transfer of heat
- Effects of heat on matter
- Relative humidity, specific heat
- Temperature scales
- Regulation of body temperature
- Use of heat for sterilization
- Application of these principles in nursing

Chapter 6

- **Light:** Laws of reflection
- Focussing elements of the eye, defective vision and its correction, use of lenses
- Relationship between energy, frequency and wavelength of light
- Biological effects of light
- Use of light in therapy
- Application of these principles in nursing

Chapter 7

- **Pressures:** Atmospheric pressure, hydrostatic pressure, osmotic pressure
- Measurements of pressures in the body:
  - Arterial and venous blood pressures
  - Ocular pressure
  - Intracranial pressure
  - Applications of these principles in nursing.

Chapter 8

- **Sound:** Frequency, velocity and intensity
- Vocalization and hearing
- Use of ultrasound. Noise pollution and its prevention
- Application of these principles in nursing.

Chapter 9

- **Electricity and Electromagnetism:** Nature of electricity. Voltage, current, resistance and their units
- Flow of electricity in solids, electrolytes, gases and vacuum
- Electricity and human body
- ECG, EEG, EMG, ECT

- Pacemakers and defibrillation
- Magnetism and electricity
- MRI scanning, CAT scan

Chapter 10

- **Atomic Energy:** Structure of atom, isotopes and isobars.
- **Radioactivity:** Use of radioactive isotopes
- Radiation protection units and limits, instruments used for detection of Ionising radiation. X-rays.

Chapter 11

- **Principles of Electronics:** Common electronic equipments used in patient care.

Practicum

- Experiments and tests should be demonstrated wherever applicable.

CHAPTER 1

Introduction to Biophysics

Suresh K Sharma, Navjot Kaur

CHAPTER OUTLINE
- Meaning of Biophysics
- Importance of Biophysics in Nursing
- Concept of Units
- Fundamental and Derived Units
- Systems of Units
- Fundamental Units in Various Systems

■ INTRODUCTION

Nature around us is colorful and full of phenomena of many varieties. The air, light, sands, water, planets, heating, electricity, functioning of the human body, there are a large number of objects and events happening around us. Physics is the study of all this. Events of nature take place according to some basic laws and knowing these basic laws from observed events is physics. Understanding physics leads to many applications in the bio and medical sciences. Biophysics is a branch of science that uses methods of physics to study biological systems.

Modern biophysics combines state-of-the-art physical measurements with computational models to understand the detailed physical mechanisms underlying the behavior of complex biological systems. Biophysics is a growing enterprise worldwide, driven primarily by the widespread realization of the major contribution that can be made to biological science by a combination of truly state-of-the-art physical measurements with modern molecular biology. The field occupies a unique and central position at the intersection of the biological, chemical, physical, and computational sciences.

Biophysics is intrinsically interdisciplinary. Biophysics takes a quantitative, physical, and non-phenomenological approach to biology that is firmly rooted in the principles of condensed phase of physics and physical chemistry. Biophysicists are driven primarily by their curiosity about how biological systems work at the molecular level. While they routinely employ the methods of molecular biology, their primary focus is on the development of novel structures and dynamical tools that enable uniquely incisive studies of systems ranging in complexity from single proteins *in vitro* to the complex interactions of biopolymers in live cells. Biophysicists as a group most often develop novel, sophisticated experimental methods that reveal molecular level details with unprecedented clarity. The state-of-the-art in X-ray crystallography, solution phase, and solid-state NMR, atomic force microscopy, single-molecule methods, EPR, and fluorescence microscopy continues to evolve in ways that better elucidate biological structure and function. In parallel, biophysicists are developing powerful new computational tools based on firmly established physical principles that are sufficiently accurate to greatly enhance insights from the experiment. Just as the tools of molecular biology gradually become useful to biophysicists, over time the new tools developed by biophysicists gradually find widespread use among all biological scientists.

■ MEANING OF BIOPHYSICS

The term biophysics was first used in 1892 by Karl Pearson in his book "The Grammar of Sciences"

- ❖ "Biophysics is defined as the science where there is the application of the laws of physics to life process".
- ❖ "Biophysics is the application of physical principles and methods to the study of the structure of living organisms and the mechanisms of the life process".
- ❖ "It is the science of living physics; the form of physics applies the knowledge of physics to explain biological questions, such as the transmission of nervous impulses or muscle control".
- ❖ "Biophysics is a branch of science that deals with the study of physical or biophysical principles and their application to health sciences".
- ❖ Biophysics is an interdisciplinary scientific discipline which uses physical techniques and methods to study the functions, structures, and energetics of biological objects.

■ IMPORTANCE OF BIOPHYSICS IN NURSING

The study of biophysics immensely benefits the nurses, because it helps them to acquire:

CHAPTER 1: Introduction to Biophysics

- Practical, functional knowledge of physical principles that underline nursing procedures and the operation of machinery that nurses use.
- Technical knowledge from the science of physics that applies specifically to nursing performance and understanding of certain biomedical phenomena, like how does a suction apparatus operate? What is the most efficient way to move a heavy object or a patient? How does air get in and out of the lungs? etc.

The study of biophysics help to understand movement, electrophysiology, membrane physics, the three-dimensional structure of proteins, protein-DNA interactions, glycoprotein structure and function, gene expression, and network theories applied to cellular metabolism and macromolecular interactions.

In addition study of biophysics helps a nurse to understand the following contents of nursing:

Measurement
- Accuracy in preparation of medications.
- Assessment of patients by measurement of vital signs

Motion
- Inertia in accidents
- The physiological reaction to high-velocity centrifuges

Gravity
- Circulation of blood
- Postural drainage
- Postoperative position
- ESR estimation
- Dependent position for edema patient

Center of Gravity
- Body mechanics
- Lifting and turning patients
- Crutch walking

Specific Gravity
- Underwater exercises
- Examination of the body fluids

Force
- Torques in traction
- Muscle action
- Vector addition and analysis in traction.

Pressure
- Suction
- Internal and external respiration
- Positive pressure ventilation
- Oxygen therapy
- Administration of irrigation and parental fluid.

Heat
- Thermometry
- Application of heat and cold application
- Steam inhalation
- Basal metabolism
- Thermography
- Autoclave and sterilization.

Light and Sound
- Actions of lenses
- Use of mirrors in apparatus
- Microscopy
- Ophthalmoscope
- Refraction
- Visual fields
- Audiometry
- Human audibility.

Electricity
- Patient monitors, ECG, EEG, EMG
- Diathermy
- Electrosurgical procedures
- Electric shock therapy
- Use of transistors in apparatus
- Cardiac pacemakers.

Work and Energy
- Circulation of blood
- Pulse formation
- Work done by heart and skeletal muscles.

Molecular Physics
- Artificial kidney
- Colloidal dispersions
- The surface tension of antiseptics
- The viscosity of blood.

Atomic Physics
- High energy radiation
- X-ray therapy
- Radioisotopes
- Tracer studies of metabolism
- Precautions in the use of radioactive material
- Half-life in radiotherapy.

■ CONCEPT OF UNITS

Nursing care demands several measurement tasks like measuring vital signs, patient's height, weight, body mass index, 24 hours fluid balance, and so many others. In this situation, a nurse takes a measurement of a physical quantity and compares the measured value of the physical quantity with a standard to determine its relationship with that standard. The standard of measurement is called a unit.

"The unit of any measurement is defined as a conventional quantity used as the reference or standard of measurement to which measurements with that unit can be compared".

■ FUNDAMENTAL AND DERIVED UNITS

Fundamental units are the units of the fundamental physical quantities in the SI system which are not formed from other units. There are a total of seven fundamental units such as meter, kilogram, ampere, and second. Derived units are those units that are used for derived quantities. Examples of derived units are meter per second (distance), mole per cubic meter (amount of substance concentration) and specific volume (cubic meter per kilogram). Total of 21 derived SI units are present. "Units of various physical quantities, which can be expressed in terms of the fundamental units of mass, length and time, are called derived units."

The unit of measurement is fixed by definition and is independent of such physical conditions as temperature, humidity, etc. The numerical value of a physical quantity, therefore, refers to the number of standard unit of measurement. For example, when we say that a patient's temperature is 38°C; it means that the patient's temperature is 38 times the unit of measurement, called degree Celsius (°C). Thus, measurement of any quantity has two characteristics—a numerical value and a unit. For example, you measure the birth weight of a baby as 3.5 Kg. Then 3.5 is the numerical value and Kg is the unit.

Although the number of physical quantities that we measure is very large, we do not need a very large number of standards to compare every measurement. It is so because all the physical

quantities are not independent quantities in so far as their measurement is concerned. For example, the velocity of a body is measured in units of length (meter) and time (seconds). A few independent standards have been chosen to fix the units of certain physical quantities. The measurement of most of the other physical quantities can be expressed in terms of these independent standards. These independent standards are length, mass and time. Such units fixed by independent standards are called fundamental units. For example, fundamental units of length, mass and time are:
- *One meter:* the unit of length
- *One kilogram:* the unit of mass
- *One second:* the unit of time

Units of measurement of many physical quantities such as density, speed, volume, pressure, and force can be derived from these fundamental or basic units using physical equations. These units are called derived units. For example, the unit of volume is a cubic meter, which is derived from the unit of length. Speed is defined as the distance covered per unit of time and its unit is m/s. The unit of speed is derived from units of length and time.

■ SYSTEMS OF UNITS

A system of units is a set of related units that are used for calculations. The system includes base units, which represent base dimensions, and derived units. There are several systems of units that have been used for measuring physical quantities. The commonly used systems are the centimeter-gram-second (CGS), the foot-pound-second (FPS), the metre-kilogram-second (MKS), and the International System of Units (SI). They differ from each other because different standards of measurement are used for fundamental quantities. **Table 1.1** contains the standards of measurement for fundamental quantities in these systems.

The two systems of measurement most frequently used in nursing practice are the MKS (also called metric) and the FPS (also called English). You may note from **Table 1.1** that the units for these physical quantities are the same in the metric and SI systems. The International System of Units (abbreviated SI) is the metric system used in science, industry, and medicine.

■ FUNDAMENTAL UNITS IN VARIOUS SYSTEMS

Units of Length

Length is defined as the distance between two points in space. The unit of length in the English system is the foot. The unit of length in

Table 1.1: Systems of units with their standards of measurement.

Physical quantity	CGS system	FPS system	MKS system	SI system
Length	Centimeter (cm)	Foot (f)	Meter (m)	Meter (m)
Mass	Gram (gm)	Pound (d)	Kilogram (kg)	Kilogram (kg)
Time	Second (s)	Second (s)	Second (s)	Second (s)
Temperature	–	Fahrenheit (F)	Celsius (°C)	Kelvin (K)
Electric current	–	–	–	Ampere (A)
Light intensity	–	–	–	Candela (Cd)
Amount of substance	–	–	–	Mole (mol)

the metric system is the meter. The bigger unit of measuring length is kilometer. Smaller measurement units are decimeter, centimeter and millimeter. The standard unit of length is 'Meter' which is written in short as 'm'.

In the health care system, one can observe the use of different systems like patient's height recorded in feet, whereas small size papule on the skin is measured in millimeters. Similarly, in microscopic work, a very small unit—a micron is used. The micron is 1/1,000 mm.

The various multiples of units of length are listed in **Table 1.2** for both metric and English systems.

The instruments used to measure length are an infantometer, measuring tape, stadiometer (measuring height)

Table 1.2: Multiples of units of length in English and metric systems.

English system	Metric system
12 inches = 1 foot	10 millimeters (mm) = 1 centimeter (cm)
3 feet = 1 yard	10 centimeters (cm) = 1 decimeter
5 ½ yards = 1 rod	10 decimeters = 1 meter (m)
1,760 yards = 1 mile	10 meters = 1 decameter
5,280 feet = 1 mile	10 decameters = 1 hectometer
	10 hectometers = 1 kilometer (km)
	10 kilometers = 1 myriameter
Note: 1 feet = 12 inches = 30 cm (1 inch = 2.5 cm)	

Unit of Mass and Weight

The mass of a body refers to the quantity of matter contained in it. The unit of mass in the metric system and SI system is the kilogram (kg). A physical balance ordinarily measures the mass of a body. **Table 1.3** shows the unit of mass in the English system and metric system. Some of these units are used in measuring food items for special diets, amount of drugs, weights of patients, etc.

Although commonly we use the terms mass and weight in the same sense, the two terms have different meanings in physics. In physics, concepts of mass and weight are different. The mass of a body is the quantity of matter contained in it. On the other hand, weight is defined as the gravitational force with which a body is pulled towards the center of the earth. Mathematically, we write:

$$W = mg$$

Where 'W' denotes the weight of the body, 'm' is its mass and 'g' is the acceleration due to gravity.

The kilogram is the SI unit of mass and it is the almost universally used standard mass unit. In the SI system, the unit of weight is Newton. 1 kilogram weighing 9.8 Newtons.

Table 1.3: Multiples of units of mass in the metric and English systems.

English system	Metric system
Troy units	10 milligrams = 1 centigram
24 grains = 1 pennyweight	
20 pennyweights = 1 ounce	10 centigrams = 1 decigram
12 ounces = 1 pound	
Avoirdupois units	10 decigrams = 1 gram
27.34 grains = 1 dram	
16 drams = 1 ounce	10 grams = 1 decagram
16 ounces = 1 pound	
25 pounds = 1 quarter	
4 quarters = 1 hundredweight	
20 hundredweights = 1 shorts ton	10 decagrams = 1 hectogram
2,240 pounds = 1 long ton	10 hectograms = 1 kilogram
Apothecaries unit	1,000 kilograms = 1 metric ton
20 grains = 1 scruple	
3 scruples = 1 dram	
8 drams = 1 ounce	
12 ounces = 1 pound	

CHAPTER 1: Introduction to Biophysics

Since the value of the acceleration due to gravity varies with the distance of an object from the center of the earth, the weight of the object changes with its position on the earth. For example, an object at sea level weighs more than it does on a high mountain because the value of the acceleration due to the gravity of the earth on the object is greater at sea level. The mass, however, remains the same everywhere. The mass of an object is measured by a physical balance, whereas its weight is measured by a spring balance.

Mass is a scalar quantity while weight is a vector quantity because it is directed toward the center of the earth. The mass of a person is the same on the earth as well as on the moon, but the weight of the person is different in these two places because their pulls on the person are different. A person weighs six times more on earth than on the moon.

Whereas mass and weight have the same numerical value, it is important in solving problems to indicate the unit specifically, as one of force (weight) or as one of mass. One gram (gm) is a unit of mass; one gram weight is a unit of weight **(Table 1.4)**.

Table 1.4: Conversion of weight and measurements.

Weight	Fluid volume
1 ounce = 8 drams	60 minims = 1 fluid dram
12 ounces = 1 pound	8 fluid drams = 1 fluid ounce
1000 micrograms (mcg) = 1 milligram (mg)	20 fluid ounces = 1 pint
1000 milligrams (mg) = 1 gram (gm)	2 pints = 1 quart (1000 ml)
1000 grams (g) = 1 kilogram (kg)	8 pints = 1 gallon
1 kilogram (kg) = 2.2 pounds	1 milliliters (ml) = 15–16 minims (15–16 drops)
1 grain = 60 milligrams (mg)	1 liter = 35 fluid ounce
1 dram = 4 grams (g)	1 fluid ounce = 30 ml
	1 fluid dram = 4 ml
1 ounce = 30 grams	1 gallon = 4.5 liters
1 pound = 375 grams	1 minimus = 0.04 ml = 1 drop
1 milligram = 1/60 grains (gr)	1 pint = 500 ml
	Household measurements
	1 teaspoonful = 4 or 5 ml = 1 fluid dram = 60 drops

Units of Time

Time is defined as the continued progress of existence in the past, present and future. The unit of time is the second and is based on the natural clock. The natural clock is governed by the time taken by the earth to complete one revolution around the moon. According to this clock, one second is defined as (1/86,400) part of a mean solar day; a solar day is a period between noon of two consecutive days, and a mean solar day is the average solar day over a year, which is 24 hours. Since one hour contains 60 minutes and one minute contains 60 seconds, a mean solar day of 24 hours would have 24 × 60 × 60 = 86,400. Thus, one second is 1/86400th part of a mean solar day.

Let us consider some of the measurements of time you make in the course of your work. You will see that the second's hand of your watch is sufficiently accurate for recording a patient's pulse rate (number of pulse beats per minute). However, for studying the heartbeat of a patient by electrocardiography, greater accuracy in the measurement of time is required. In this case, the beating of the heart must be accurately measured in tenths or hundredths of a second.

Table 1.5 lists some of the prefixes and symbols used with SI and metric units to express a very large or very small value:

Table 1.5: Prefixes and symbols used with SI units and metric units.			
Prefix	Symbol	Power	Value
Tera	T	10^{12}	1,000,000,000,000
Giga	G	10^{9}	1,000,000,000
Mega	M	10^{6}	1,000,000
Kilo	K	10^{3}	1,000
Hecto	H	10^{2}	100
Deca	Da	10	10
Meter	M	1	1
Deci	D	10^{-1}	.1
Centi	C	10^{-2}	.01
Milli	Mm	10^{-3}	.001
Micro	U	10^{-6}	.000001
Nano	N	10^{-9}	.000000001
Pico	P	10^{-12}	.000000000001
Femto	F	10^{-15}	.000000000000001
Atto	A	10^{-18}	.000000000000000001

CHAPTER 1: Introduction to Biophysics

Table 1.6: Conversion between metric and English systems.

Weight	Length	Volume
1 gram = 15 grains	2.54 centimeters = 1 inch	1 cubic centimeter = 15 minims
4 grams = 1 dram	1 meter = 39.37 inches	4 cubic centimeters = 1 fluid dram
30 grams = 1 ounce		30 cubic centimeters = 1 fluid ounce
454 grams = 1 pound		
1 kilogram = 2.2 pounds		

In nursing practice, one may come across situations when a measurement is taken in the metric unit must be changed to the corresponding English unit and vice versa. For this reason, approximate equivalents commonly used in the hospital are given in **Table 1.6**.

■ QUESTIONS

Q.1: Discuss the meaning and importance of biophysics in nursing.
Q.2: Discuss the concept of units and fundamental and derived units.
Q.3: Describe the different systems of the units.
Q.4: List out the basic units of length, weight, mass, and time.

■ BIBLIOGRAPHY

1. Cantor CR, Schimmel PR. Biophysical Chemistry, Volumes 1–3. WH Freeman, San Francisco, 1980.
2. Cantor CR, Schimmel PR. Biophysical Chemistry, Volumes 1–3. WH Freeman, San Francisco, 1980.
3. Cotterill RMJ. Biophysics: An Introduction, Wiley, 2002.
4. Cotterill RMJ. Biophysics: An Introduction, Wiley, 2002.
5. Dogonadze RR, Urushadze ZD. "Semi-Classical Method of Calculation of Rates of Chemical Reactions Proceeding in Polar Liquids". J Electroanal Chem, 1971; 32: 235–45.
6. Flitter HH, Rowe HR. An Introduction to Physics in Nursing. St Louis: The CV Mosby Company, 1995.
7. Glaser R. Biophysics, Springer, 2001.
8. Glaser R. Biophysics: An Introduction (Corrected Edition). Springer, 2004: 11-23.
9. Glaser R. Biophysics: An Introduction. Springer Verlag, Heidelberg, 2004.
10. 10 Gomber KL, Gogia KL. Fundamental Physics. Ambala: Publishers, 2004.

11. Goyal RP, Tripathi SP. Concise Physics. New Delhi: Selina Publishers, August 2007.
12. Hobbie RK, Roth BJ. Intermediate Physics for Medicine and Biology (4th Edition). Springer, 2006.
13. Hobbie RK, Roth BJ. International Physics for Medicine and Biology (4th Edition). Springer, 2006.
14. Jackson B. Molecular and cellular biophysics. New York: Cambridge Publication, 2006.
15. Lal S. Principles of Physics. Ambala: Paedeep Publishers, 2004.
16. Mielczarek VE, Greenbaum E, et al. Biological Physics. New York. American Institute of Physics, 1993.
17. Nelson PC. Biological Physics (Updated Edition). WH Freeman, 2007.
18. Perutz MF. "The haemoglobin molecule". Proceedings of the Royal Society of London. Series, 1969;B 173(31)113-40.
19. Perutz MF. Electrostatic Effects in Proteins, Science. 1978;201:1187-91.
20. Perutz MF. Proteins and Nucleic Acids, Elsevier, Amsterdam, 1962.
21. Perutz MF. Proteins and Nucleic Acids: Structure and Function. Amsterdam: Elsevier, 1962.
22. Phillips R, Kondev J, Theriot J. Physical Biology of the Cell. Garland Science, Oxford, 2008.
23. Rashevsky N. Mathematical biophysics. Rev. ed., University of Chicago Press, 1948.
24. Rashevsky N. Mathematical Biophysics: Physico- Mathematical Foundations of Biology - Vol.2, New York: Dover Publications, Third Revised Edition, 1960.
25. Ruch TC, Fulton JF. Medical Physiology and Biophysics. Saunders, 1974: 1232.
26. Sneppen K, Zocchi G. Physics in Molecular Biology, Cambridge University Press, 2005.
27. Sneppen K, Zocchi G. Physics in Molecular Biology, First edition. Cambridge University Press, 2005:10-7.
28. Volkenshtein MV, Dogonadze RR, Madumarov AK, et al. Theory of Enzyme Catalysis. Molekuliarnaya Biologia (Moscow)1972; 6: 431-9 (In Russian, English summary).
29. Biophysics in nursing education. AIP Conference Proceedings 2152, 030019 (2019); https://doi.org/10.1063/1.5124763
30. Miroslava Líšková, Ľubomíra Valovičová, and Ján Ondruška. Collection Development Guidelines of the National Library of Medicine [Internet]. Bethesda (MD): National Library of Medicine (US); 2019-. Biophysics. [Updated 2004 Jan 2]. Available from: https://www.ncbi.nlm.nih.gov/sites/books/NBK518712/

CHAPTER 2

Motion

Suresh K Sharma, Navjot Kaur

Chapter Outline
- Scalars and Vectors
- Rest and Motion
- Speed
- Velocity
- Acceleration
- Applications of Motion in Nursing

■ INTRODUCTION

Motion is such an important phenomenon that life cannot be imagined without it. In physics, motion is the phenomenon in which an object changes its position over time. Motion is mathematically described in terms of displacement, distance, velocity, acceleration, speed, and time. The motion of the earth around the Sun gives rise to different seasons and the earth's motion on its own axis results in the occurrence of day and night. Most of the human body functions cannot be accomplished without motion, as the motion of the heart helps in pumping the blood in the body. Breathing is also only possible with the motion of the lungs. Similarly, there are several other body functions or activities of human life, where motion is essential to accomplish them, like transfer of a patient from bed to chair or administration of blood or fluid is only possible with the existence of the phenomenon of motion.

To understand the concept of motion, it is important to be familiar with scalar and vector quantities:

■ SCALARS AND VECTORS

- **Scalar quantities:** The physical quantities, which have a magnitude (how much) but no direction, are called scalars. For example, mass,

Table 2.1: Difference between a vector and scalar quantity.

	Vector	Scalar
Definition	A physical quantity with both the magnitude and direction	A physical quantity with only magnitude.
Representation	A number (magnitude), direction using unit cap or arrow at the top and unit	A number (magnitude) and unit
Symbol	Quantity symbol in bold and an arrow sign above	Quantity symbol
Direction	Yes	No
Example	Velocity and acceleration	Mass and temperature

length, temperature, work, charge, specific heat, time, density, etc. It may be positive or negative.

❖ **Vector quantities:** The physical quantities, which possess both magnitude and direction (which way), are called vectors. For example, displacement, velocity, acceleration, force, weight, momentum, etc.

To appreciate the difference between a scalar quantity and a vector quantity **(Table 2.1)**, suppose that an ambulance picks up a patient from a point "X" and travels along a path shown by the dashed curve and arrives at the hospital at point "P". The distance traveled by the ambulance is the total length of the dashed line, irrespective of the direction in which it travels. The curved line "XP" is 10.5 cm long. This is the value of the distance covered by the ambulance. Note that, in this case, the direction along which the ambulance travels is not important. That is why we say that distance is a scalar quantity. It has magnitude but no direction. Further, as mentioned above displacement is the shortest distance between the initial and the final positions. Thus, in **Fig. 2.1**, the straight line "XP" (= 9 cm) represents

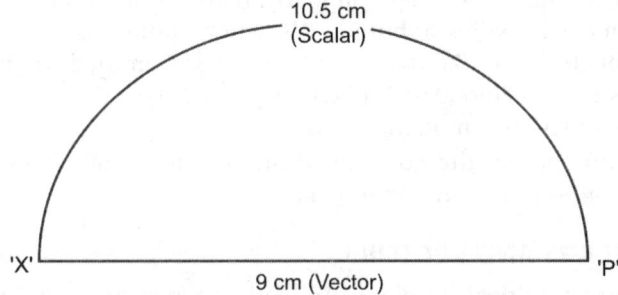

Fig. 2.1: Scalar and vector quantity.

the displacement and the direction of displacement is along "XP". Displacement, therefore, is a vector quantity and has magnitude as well as direction. From the knowledge of the distance covered by the vehicle, we may form an idea about the petrol consumed but we cannot locate the vehicle. For this we must know its displacement from a certain location.

Therefore, here total distance covered by ambulance is a scalar quantity and displacement of ambulance for 'X' place to 'P' is vector quantity.

■ REST AND MOTION

There are two states of objects in physics i.e. Rest and motion. While traveling in a train, you find that your co-passenger is at rest but the viewer on ground tells that person is moving. The book in your hands is at rest if viewed from the room and is moving if viewed from moon. When we say an object is moving or is at rest... what exactly do we mean?

Motion is a combined property of the body under observation and observer. There is no meaning of rest and motion without a viewer. The viewer on ground is moving with respect to the train and train is moving with respect to that person. The moon is moving with respect to the book and the book is moving with respect to the moon.

From the above discussion, we can conclude if a body changes its position with respect to the viewer as time passes, it is said to be in motion and if it does not change its position, then it is at rest.

Motion is defined as "An act of change in position of an object with time with respect to some fixed position, which is taken as the reference point".

If an object or subject changes its position in reference to a fixed point with a time interval, it is said to be in motion. Basically, motion is a result of the force. One may experience several kinds of forces in day-to-day life to have motion. Such as muscular force causes blood circulation of the body or movement of lungs results in respiration. Gravitational forces contribute toward motion of fluids; therefore administration of nasogastric feed or intravenous fluids can be possible. Several other examples of motion like walking, exercise, lifting a load all the activities need some or other kind of force.

Types of Motion

In physics, motion is classified into various categories:
- ❖ **Translatory motion:** It is also called as linear motion. Motion in a straight path is named as translatory motion like walking.

- **Circular motion:** In a circular motion, the object just moves in a circle. The revolution of the earth around the sun, artificial satellites going around the Earth at a constant height.Movements of the magnetic fields around the body parts of the patient during Magnetic Resonance Imaging (MRI) or rotation of test tubes in a centrifuge are the another good examples for circular motion.
- **Rotational motion:** The object rotates about an axis, e.g., earth rotating on its own axis.
- **Oscillatory motion:** Something that oscillates moves back and forth. Anything that repeats the motion cycle after a certain period is considered to be oscillating. The pendulum of the clock oscillates about a point. In process of breathing, lungs move inside the chest in oscillatory manner. Similarly our intestines exhibit rhythmic motion as they move food towards its final destination.

Primarily the motion of objects can be studied under two separate headings:
- **Kinematics:** The study of the motion of the objects without taking into account the cause of their motion is called kinematics.
- **Dynamics:** The study of the motion of the objects by taking into account the cause(s) of their change of state is called dynamics. For example, gas molecules are always in causeless random motion, though their motion is not visible to the naked eye.

■ SPEED

Speed is a scalar quantity. Speed refers to the distance traveled by an object in a particular interval of time and is defined as a measure of distance covered in a time limit. In other words the time rate of covering the distance by a particle is called its speed. Consider the flow of blood inside our bodies. Its flowthrough capillaries is very slow, whereas, in larger vessels, it moves relatively rapidly. To quantify such observations, we define a physical parameter called speed as the rate of change of distance with time. Mathematically.

$$\text{Speed} = \frac{\text{Distance}}{\text{Time}}$$

The SI unit for speed is meter per second (ms^{-1}). The unit of speed is derived from the unit of length and unit of time. Speed indicates how fast a body is moving and does not specify the direction along which the body is moving.

■ VELOCITY

The physical parameter, which specifies how fast a body is moving and in which direction it is moving is called the velocity of the body.

CHAPTER 2: Motion

Thus, velocity is a vector quantity. The velocity of an object is the rate of change of its position with respect to a frame of reference, and is a function of time

Speed of the object in a particular direction. Mathematically, we write

$$\text{Velocity} = \frac{\text{Displament}}{\text{Time}}$$

The SI unit of velocity is the same as that of speed. But it is expressed with direction (because it is a vector quantity), for example, 50 ms^{-1} from A to B, or 50 ms^{-1} eastwards. Generally, in real-life situations, the direction is understood according to the situation and not expressed explicitly.

Types of Velocity

- **Uniform velocity:** An object is said to be moving with uniform velocity, if it undergoes equal displacements in equal intervals of time, however small these intervals of time may be.
- **Variable velocity:** An object is said to be moving with variable velocity, if either its speed or its direction of motion or both change with time.
- **Average velocity:** The ratio of total change in position or displacement to the total time taken is called average speed.
- **Instantaneous velocity:** The velocity of an object at a particular instant of time or at a particular point of its path is called the instantaneous velocity of the object.

■ ACCELERATION

Another useful physical parameter that specifies a change in velocity with time is called acceleration. It is defined as follows:

The rate of increase in speed is known as acceleration. In other words "the time rate of change of velocity of an object is called the acceleration of the object". The object is said to be moving with constant acceleration and such a motion is called uniformly accelerated motion.

The SI unit of acceleration is ms^{-2}. An example of accelerated motion is the flow of blood inside the human body, which circulates in different parts with different velocities. Acceleration, like velocity, is a vector quantity. Acceleration is regarded as positive if the velocity is increasing with time. A decreasing velocity refers to negative acceleration and it is usually called deceleration.

You can visualize the blood flow from arteries to the capillaries as deceleration and from capillaries to the heart as acceleration.

Types of Accelerations

Average acceleration: An object's average acceleration over a period of time is its change, divided by the duration of the period.

Instantaneous acceleration: Acceleration at a specific instant of time.

■ APPLICATIONS OF MOTION IN NURSING

With study of motion, nurses will be able to understand:

Motion during Walking

Walking is energy efficient. In a walking human, one leg swings forward while the other leg's foot stays planted on the ground. When walking at natural speed (defined below), the swinging leg uses muscle force to move forward and immediately relaxes, allowing the force of gravity to move it to the ground. Simultaneously, the planted leg moves forward with largely passive rotation at the hip. The plant leg only needs to stay straight and the swinging leg's knee only slightly bends to allow it to pass underneath the body. We have difficulty in walking on wet surface due to less friction and labored walking on sand which is having high friction.

So condition of floor and footwear of patient should be kept in mind while moving the patient and there should be enough friction for smooth walking and maintaining gait.

Motion Sickness

During the movement of body endolymph moves in inner ear and our balance is maintained by input from vision, nerves of the muscles and joints, and the vestibular system (inner ear) which is processed into meaningful information by the central vestibular system (brainstem). When movements are jerky and in rotational manner fluid moves in same direction due to inertia but the body is either stationary or moving in another direction so contradictory inputs from vision and vestibular system result in the sensations of dizziness, vertigo, or disequilibrium and this can be treated by medication or by Epley maneuver or Brandt-Daroff exercise.

Motion in Centrifuge Devices

A centrifuge is a metal rotor with holes to accommodate vessels of liquid, spun at selected speeds by a motor. Low-speed centrifuges generally operate at up to 10,000 revolutions per minute (rpm) and may be non-refrigerated or refrigerated. High-speed centrifuges generally operate at 10,000–30,000 rpm and some are refrigerated to cool the rotor chamber.

Centrifuges apply centrifugal (outward pushing) force to separate suspended particles from a liquid or to separate liquids of different densities. These liquids can include body fluids (e.g., blood, serum, urine), commercial reagents, or combinations of the two with other additives. By creating forces many times greater than gravity, centrifuges can greatly accelerate separations that occur naturally as a result of density differences. The applications includes study of viruses, proteins, nucleic acids, polymers and blood.

Motion and Orthostatic Hypotension

Normally, the gravitational stress of sudden standing causes 500 mL to 800 mL of blood to pool in the veins of the legs and trunk. That leads to a decrease in venous return which reduces cardiac output and thus BP. In the response to this fall in BP, baroreceptors in the aortic arch and carotid sinus activate autonomic reflexes to rapidly return the BP to normal. The sympathetic nervous system increases heart rate and contractility and increases the vasomotor tone of the capacitance vessels. Simultaneous parasympathetic (vagal) inhibition also increases heart rate. In most people, changes in BP and heart rate upon standing are minimal and transient, and symptoms do not occur. But nurses should be cautious in moving an old age person and the person who was on bed for long period, out of bed. Because they are prone to develop orthostatic hypotension. This should also be kept in mind while moving the patient through lifts.

Health implications of high velocity motion vehicles like airplanes and rockets where a person moving in a highly accelerated vehicle is known as acceleration stress.

Inertia in Accidents

According to law of inertia if a body is moving it remains in motion unless external force is applied, during accident body remains in speed even after vehicle stopped so due to this, a person remaining in vehicle without seat belt may have severe injuries hitting himself with body of the vehicle and due to jerk, there may be a fracture in the spine without external injury.

According to the definition, force is equal to the rate of change in momentum with time ($F = m \times v/t$) showing that if time is reduced then force will be increased. Using this principle karate player can break tiles with a high speed hand and if during accident, time of collision is less, then injury will be severe even with a light vehicle. So for assessment during road traffic accident special precaution should be given to spine and head.

■ QUESTIONS

Q.1: Discuss the types of motion.
Q.2: Explain the application of principles of the motion in nursing.
Q.3: A fast moving wheelchair on which a patient is sitting should not be stopped suddenly, discuss.

■ BIBLIOGRAPHY

1. Bowen R. Gastrointestinal Transit: How Long Does It Take? Colorado State University, 2006.
2. David H, George H, Keith B. "Velocity and Drag Forces on motor-protein-driven Vesicles in Cells". American Physical Society, the 69th Annual Meeting of the Southeastern, 2002.
3. Fischer M, Franzeck UK, Herrig I. "Flow velocity of single lymphatic capillaries in human skin". Am J Physiol Heart Circ Physiology, 1996; 270.
4. Hubble E. "A Relation between Distance and Radial Velocity among Extra-Galactic Nebulae" Proceedings of the National Academy of Sciences of the United States of America, 1929;15 (3), 1929: 168-73.
5. Kogut A, Lineweaver C, Smoot GF, et al. Dipole Anisotropy in the COBE Differential Microwave Radiometers First- Year Sky Maps. Astrophysical Journal, 1993; 419: 1.
6. Meschede M, Udo Barckhausen U. (November 20, 2000). "Plate Tectonic Evolution of the Cocos-Nazca Spreading Center". Proceedings of the Ocean Drilling Program. Texas A and M University. http://www-odp.tamu.edu/publications/170_SR/chap_07/chap_07. htm Retrieved, 2007: 04-02.
7. Nave R. Motion HyperPhysics. Georgia State University, 2005.
8. Newton's. "Axioms or Laws of Motion" can be found in the "Principia" volume-1, 1729: 19.
9. Penny P. Hemodynamic: Blood Velocity, 2003.
10. Safkan Y. "The term 'absolute motion' has no meaning, then why do we say that the earth moves around the sun and not vice versa?" Ask the Experts. Physics Link, 2007.
11. Tyson DG, Liu NC, Irion R. One Universe: At home in the cosmos. Joseph Henry Press, 2000.
12. Wahlin L. "THE DEADBEAT UNIVERSE". Chapter 9. Colutron Research Corporation, 1997.
13. Kiseleva TA, Klochkov YV, Nikolaev AP. Comparison of scalar and vector FEM forms in the case of an elliptic cylinder. Comput. Math. and Math. Phys. 2015;55:422–31. https://doi.org/10.1134/S0965542515030094

CHAPTER 3

Gravity

Suresh K Sharma, Navjot Kaur

Chapter Outline
- Specific Gravity
- Center of Gravity
- Principles of Gravity
- Mass and Weight
- Effects of Gravitational Forces on Human Body and Applications of Principles of Gravity in Nursing

■ INTRODUCTION

Gravity is defined as the accelerating tendency of the bodies toward the center of the earth or towards the center of the other heavenly bodies, such as the moon. Gravity is very important to us. We could not live on Earth without it. The sun's gravity keeps Earth in orbit around it, keeping us at a comfortable distance to enjoy the sun's light and warmth. It holds down our atmosphere and the air we need to breathe. Gravity is what holds our world together. Gravitation is the force with which all bodies in the universe attract one another. According to Newton's law of universal gravitation, the gravitational force between any two bodies in the universe is proportional to the product of their masses and inversely proportional to the square of the distance between them.

$$F = \frac{G M_1 M_2}{d^2}$$

Where,
F = gravitational force
M_1 and M_2 = any two masses in the universe
d = distance between two masses
G = universal gravitational constant = 6.67×10^{-11} Nm^2/Kg^2

■ SPECIFIC GRAVITY

Specific gravity is the ratio of the density of any substance to that of water at a specified temperature. It is also known as relative density and clinically expressed as specific gravity. Specific gravity actually signifies how many times lighter or heavier a substance is than an equal volume of water.

$$\text{Specific density} = \frac{\text{Density of the object}}{\text{Density of the water}}$$

It is common to use the density of water at 4 °C as a reference point, as water at this point has the highest density of 1000 kg/m³. The specific gravity of a substance is expressed numerically by the values of its density in grams per cubic centimeter (gm/cm³), but with the unit omitted. For example, the specific gravity of a substance 'A' with a density of 5 gm/cm³ will be 5. It means the substance is five times heavier than water under the same circumstances.

It is clear that specific gravity depends on the density of the substance; for example, if urine is concentrated and has more salts dissolved, will likely have higher specific gravity and if urine is less concentrated then specific gravity will be likely to be lower (Normal specific gravity of urine is 1.010–1.030). Similarly, the specific gravity of blood ranges between 1.055 and 1.066; blood with higher plasma proportion in comparison to blood cells will have lower specific gravity.

As we have learned that specific gravity is the ratio of the density of any substance to that of water. So to determine the specific gravity of a solid substance when weight the substance in air and then water **(Table 3.1)**. The difference between the two weights gives the

Table 3.1: Specific gravity of some substances.

Substance	Density (kg/m²)	Relative density/Specific gravity
Pure water	1000	1.00
Alcohol	790	0.79
Whole blood	1060	1.06
Blood plasma	1030	1.03
Aluminum	2700	2.70
Platinum	21400	21.40
Lead	11400	11.40
Gold	19300	19.30
Iron	7950	7.90
Mercury	13550	11.55

apparent loss of weight in water. The apparent loss of weight is equal to the weight of water displaced. Therefore, in physical properties, specific gravity can also be estimated by the following formula.

$$\text{Specific gravity} = \frac{\text{Weight of the object in air}}{\text{Weight of equal volume of water}}$$

■ CENTER OF GRAVITY

The center of gravity is considered to be the point at which all external forces are applied to an object. If an object is suspended from this point, it will remain in balance without turning whatever its position is.

In general, the center of gravity or center of mass of a body is the point at which all the mass is considered to be centered.

When a person is standing, her/his center of gravity is located in the pelvic cavity. A line drawn perpendicularly downwards from the center of gravity of a person passes through the area bounded by her/his feet **(Fig. 3.1)**. It is for this reason that while carrying a heavy object, balance is obtained easily if the feet are placed farther apart.

In nursing practice, it is often necessary for a nurse to carry heavy objects close to the body, so that the center of gravity does not deviate and does not put extra strain on the body. For example, carrying a large water basin in hands away from the body will put extra strain on back muscles since a heavy object in the hands adds weight to

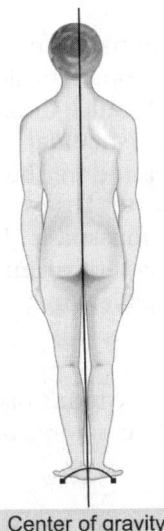

Center of gravity

Fig. 3.1: Center of gravity in a person standing.

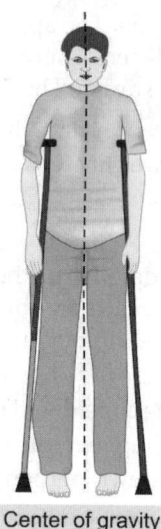

Fig. 3.2: Center of gravity in a person using crutches.

the front of the body, the center of gravity shifts forward; in order to keep the normal position and maintain equilibrium, muscles of the back exert a backward pull. To minimize this strain, one should keep the object in hand as close to the body as possible, i.e. as close to the center of gravity as possible.

For Example
- In folding a blanket, the arms should be held relaxed at the side of the body and forearms should be flexed because outstretched extremities increase the distance through which the force act on the center of rotation at the shoulder.
- During the use of crutches, the area bounded by the crutches and the uninjured foot becomes the base through which the vertical line through its center of mass must pass. These supports must be kept far enough apart so that the vertical line always passes through the base area, otherwise, the patient may fall **(Fig. 3.2)**.

■ MASS AND WEIGHT

Although commonly we use the terms mass and weight in the same sense, the two terms have different meanings in physics. In physics concepts of mass and weight are different. The mass of a body is the quantity of matter contained in it. Everything we see around us has mass. For example, a table, a chair, your bed, a football, a glass, and even air has mass. That being said, all objects are light or heavy because of their mass.

The SI unit of mass is the kilogram (kg). The formula of mass can be written as:

$$\text{Mass} = \text{Density} \times \text{Volume}$$

On the other hand, weight is defined as the gravitational force with which a body is pulled towards the center of the earth.

Mathematically, we write

$$W = mg$$

where 'W' denotes the weight of the body, 'm' is its mass and 'g' is the acceleration due to gravity.

Since the value of the acceleration due to gravity varies with the distance of an object from the center of the earth, the weight of the object changes with its position on the earth. For example, an object at sea level weighs more than it does on a high mountain because the value of the acceleration due to the gravity of the earth on the object is greater at sea level. The mass, however, remains the same everywhere.

The mass of an object is measured by a physical balance, whereas its weight is measured by a spring balance.

Mass is a scalar quantity while weight is a vector quantity because it is directed toward the center of the earth.

The mass of a person is the same on the earth as well as on the moon, but the weight of the person is different in these two places because their pulls on the person are different. A person weighs six times more on earth than on the moon.

Whereas mass and weight have the same numerical value, it is important in solving problems to indicate the unit specifically, as one of force (weight) or as one of mass.

One gram (gm) is a unit of mass.

One gram weight is unit of weight.

Mass		Weight	
Definition	Mass is defined as the amount of matter in a substance	Weight is defined as the amount of force acting on the mass of an object because of acceleration due to gravity.	
Denotation	Mass is represented by "M."	Weight is represented by "W."	
Formula	• Mass is always constant for a body. • One way to calculate mass: Mass = density × volume.	• Weight is the measure of the gravitational force acting on a mass. • Formula of weight: Weight = mass × acceleration due to gravity	
Unit of measurement	The SI unit of mass is "kilogram".	The SI unit of weight is Newton (N).	
Quantity type	• Mass is a base quantity. • Mass only has magnitude and hence, it is a scalar quantity	• Weight is a derived quantity. • Weight has both magnitude and direction (toward the center of gravity) and hence, it is a vector quantity.	
Measuring instrument	Mass can be easily measured using any ordinary balance. For example, beam balance, lever balance, pan balance, etc.	Weight can be measured by a spring balance or by using its formula given above.	

■ PRINCIPLES OF GRAVITY

The most important principle of gravity is Archimedes' Principle. Archimedes, a Greek mathematician gave Archimedes' Principle.

It is a common experience for all of us that while standing in water, we feel as if we are being pushed upwards by force acting from below. Similarly, balloons filled with a gas, say hydrogen, rise in the atmosphere on their own. In fact, all bodies experience an upward force when held inside a fluid.

The force of thrust is opposite to the force of gravity. When pressure is put on any fluid, the body is submerged in it, and this force is thrust. The force reduces as it goes down because of gravity and thus the body feels light. Swimming is an example of this concept.

$$\text{Thrust} = \text{Pressure} \times \text{Area}$$

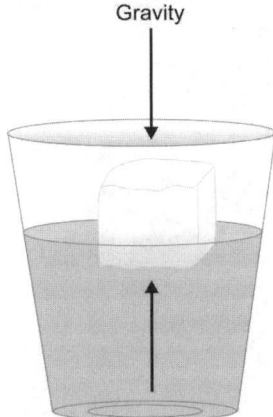

Fig. 3.3: Buoyant force.

"The tendency of a fluid to exert an upward force on an object immersed in it is called buoyancy. The upward force acting on the object is known as the buoyancy force."

The upthrust due to buoyancy results in an apparent loss in the weight of the body **(Fig. 3.3)**.

You can see its manifestation if you draw water from a well using a bucket-rope arrangement. As soon as the bucket comes out of the water, it suddenly feels heavier.

We know that when a body is immersed in a fluid, it displaces some amount of fluid. If we imagine that the space occupied by the body is replaced by the fluid, then the center of gravity of this fluid is called the center of buoyancy. The upthrust on a body acts through the center of buoyancy. If a body of uniform density is submerged fully in a fluid, then its center of gravity coincides with the center of buoyancy. The quantitative measure of buoyant force is given by Archimedes' principle.

Archimedes' principle may be stated as follows:

"When a body is wholly or partially immersed in a fluid, it experiences an upward thrust, which is equal to the weight of the fluid displaced."

This principle can also be stated as follows:
- When a body is wholly or partially immersed in a fluid, it experiences an apparent loss in its weight (due to upward thrust), which is equal to the weight of the fluid displaced by it **(Fig. 3.4)**.

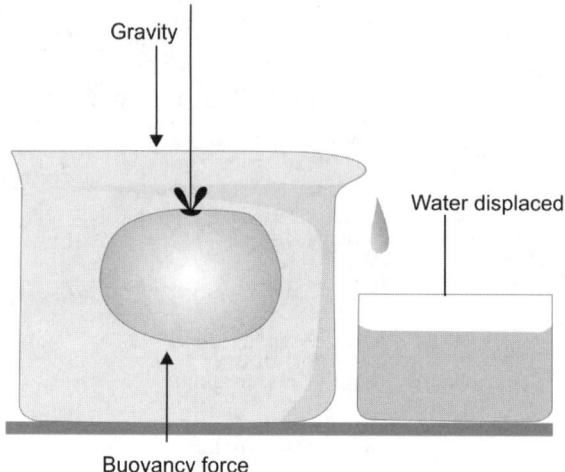

Fig. 3.4: Archimedes' Principle.

❖ Sometimes this principle is also known as the principle of buoyancy. Archimedes' principle can be used to determine the specific gravity of a solid substance.

■ APPLICATIONS OF ARCHIMEDES' PRINCIPLE

❖ Submarine – Ballast tank inside the submarine makes the weight of the submarine greater than the buoyant force.
❖ Hot air balloon – The buoyant force of a balloon is less than the surrounding air by varying the quantity of hot air in the balloon
  • A hydrometer, used for measuring the specific gravity of liquids operates on this principle.
  • Urinometer also works on the same principle.
  • Underwater exercises, where patients with joint or muscular problems can be facilitated for exercise, where they feel easy to perform exercises in water due to buoyancy forces **(Fig. 3.5)**.

■ EFFECTS OF GRAVITATIONAL FORCES ON THE HUMAN BODY AND APPLICATION OF PRINCIPLES OF GRAVITY IN NURSING

Diagnosis using principles of gravity
❖ The erythrocyte sedimentation (ESR) is based on gravity only. In this test, the sedimentation rate is measured by the depth of surface between the clear plasma and the cells in a test tube for over an hour. The faster this happens, the higher the ESR and there may be more inflammation in the body because during inflammation there

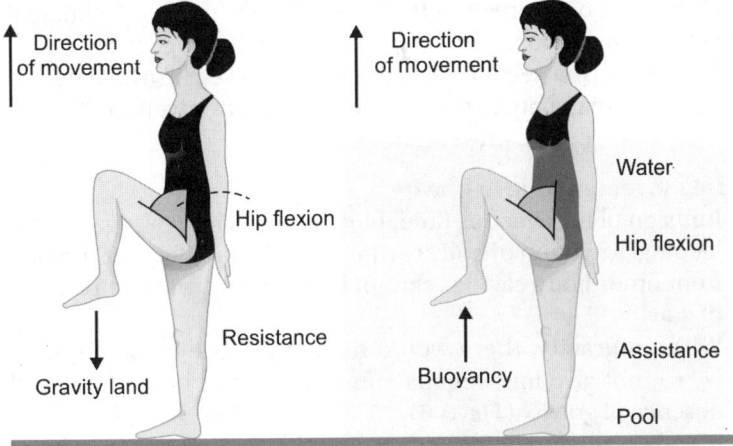

Fig. 3.5: Exercise in and out of water.

may be more protein in RBCs or they may clump together due to surface proteins and become heavier as a result more gravitational force is applied to make them settle fast.

- Haemoglobin screening is done during blood donation using an appropriately standardized $CuSO_4$ solution having a specific gravity of 1.053 based on gravitation force. If the drop of blood float on the surface it is assumed the person is having Hb level below 12 g/dl so he or she is not fit for blood donation. This is very useful during blood donation camps.
- A urine-specific gravity test compares the density of urine to the density of water by using principles of gravity. This quick test can help determine how well kidneys are diluting or concentrate the urine.

Position of the patient according to principles of gravity
- Brain surgery is frequently done with the patient in a sitting or semi-sitting position to lessen the danger of haemorrhage.
- After a rib resection, the patient is kept in a semi-sitting position to increase drainage from the thorax through the drainage tube by gravity.
- When a patient who is under the effect of anesthesia or an unconscious patient, his or her head is placed on one side, then tongue and oral secretions drop down due to gravity that makes a larger passageway for air to enter and respiration will improve.
- A dependent position with legs dragged on one side of beds, for a patient with congestive cardiac failure, it accumulate excess fluid in legs and facilitate breathing (also achieved through gravity).

- Oscillating beds are used to change the positions to facilitate the circulation of blood and lymph is achieved with gravity.
- Post radical mastectomy affected sidearm is kept in a high position, so that with gravity lymph can be drained effectively and swelling on the arm can be prevented.

Fluid movement due to gravity
- Infusion of intravenous fluid, blood transfusion, nasogastric tube feeding, irrigation of body cavities, urinary drainage, or drainages from other body cavities cannot be imagined without principles of gravity.
- Without gravity, there would be no pressure in the liquid. So we cannot give intravenous infusion or blood transfusion in the absence of gravity **(Fig. 3.6)**.
- Blood circulation in the body mainly depends on gravity. Changes in body position alter the pressure of blood in different parts of the body. If a person faints, his head should be lowered. This helps the blood to return to the head (by gravity).
- A person standing for a long period of time may have edema of the legs **(Fig. 3.7)**. Gravity exercises are sometimes prescribed for patients with circulatory disorders of the lower extremities.
- During thoracentesis, Paracentesis, the peritoneal dialysis fluid is drained with principles of gravity.
- Postural drainage after the chest physiotherapy is also based on gravity only.

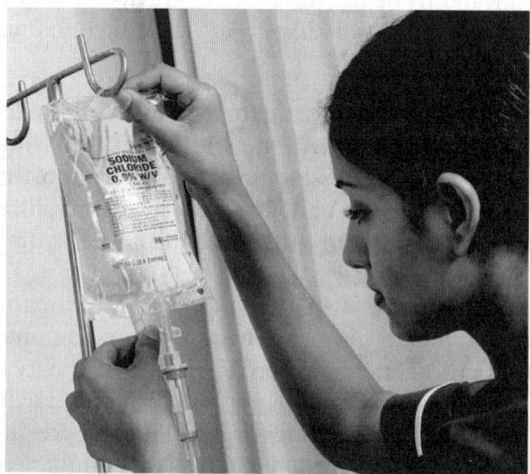

Fig. 3.6: IV fluid administration with gravity.

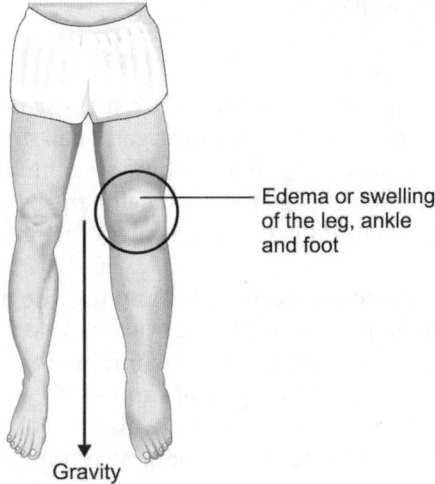

Fig. 3.7: Edema due to gravity.

Stability and gravity
Body alignment is achieved by placing one body part in line with another body part in a vertical or horizontal line. Correct alignment contributes to body balance and decreases strain on muscle-skeletal structures. Without this balance, the risk of falls and injuries increases. In the language of body mechanics, the **center of gravity** is the center of the weight of an object or person. A lower center of gravity increases stability. This can be achieved by bending the knees and bringing the center of gravity closer to the base of support, keeping the back straight. A wide base of support is the foundation for stability. A wide **base of support** is achieved by placing feet a comfortable, shoulder-width distance apart. When a vertical line falls from the center of gravity through the wide base of support, **body balance** is achieved. If the vertical line moves outside the base of support, the body will lose balance.

❖ Persons with obesity may have a greater risk of falling while walking or running because some timeline of gravity may fall out base of support, so we should be careful while moving the obese patient.

❖ Chronic low back pain may be due to having the center of gravity located excessively towards the back caused by decreased low back strength and decreased amount of normal low back curve. If center of gravity is too far, a black person might have strength and balance challenges to overcome in order to re-establish postural control. So the right posture should be maintained during the working and shifting of patients.

Patient handling and gravity

Principles of body mechanics should be applied properly during all patient-handling activities.

- ❖ Assess the weight of the load before lifting and determine if assistance is required. Plan the move; gather all supplies and clear the area of obstacles. Avoid stretching, reaching, and twisting, which may place the line of gravity outside the base of support.
- ❖ Tighten abdominal, gluteal, and leg muscles in anticipation of the move.
- ❖ Stand up straight to protect the back and provide balance.
- ❖ Place the weight of the object being moved close to your center of gravity for balance. Equilibrium is maintained as long as the line of gravity passes through its base of support.
- ❖ Facing the direction prevents abnormal twisting of the spine. Turning, rolling, pivoting, and leveraging requires less work than lifting.
- ❖ Do not lift if possible; use mechanical lifts as required.
- ❖ Encourage the patient to help as much as possible.
- ❖ Keep all work at waist level to avoid stooping. Do not bend at the waist.
- ❖ Reduce friction between surfaces so that less force is required to move the patient. Bending the knees maintain your center of gravity and let the strong muscles of your legs do the lifting.
- ❖ It is easier to push an object than to pull it.
- ❖ Less energy is required to keep an object moving than it is to stop and start it.
- ❖ Use assistive devices (gait belt, slider boards, mechanical lifts) as required to position patients and transfer them from one surface to another.
- ❖ The person with the heaviest load should coordinate all the effort of the others involved in the handling technique.

A new horizon of gravity used in medical treatment:

Neural plasticity, the ability of the brain to learn from experience and to adapt to new environments is recognized to be profound and exposure to altered gravity has an effect on communication sites between the sensory cells and the nerve fibers ending on them. This could lead to the assumption that similar exposure to a force greater than 1G on a centrifuge on earth might one day prove useful in restoring a sense of balance to disabled people who have lost it. There are cases of children with medical disorders, such as autism, attention deficit disorders, fragile X etc.

A newborn baby whose brain is damaged at birth, like in the case of cerebral palsy, may require hypergravity, a higher intensity of gravity stimulus, before a child's brain becomes programed to respond to direction and acceleration and eventually learn to walk. Increasing gravity could modify or alter his perception of it prior to responding, by triggering gravity sensors and the brain blood flow. This would mean that rehabilitation exercises in children with cerebral palsy should be more effective if done in the upright position in a way that the body may experience some load, even if the child had to be supported by a harness. Alternately, the movement therapy could be done on a centrifuge.

■ QUESTIONS

Q.1: The point where the whole weight of the body may be supposed to act is called as......................
Q.2: Hydrometer works on the principle of ....
Q.3: Back should be kept upright while carrying a tray; why explain?
Q.4: What is the principle of lactometer in measuring specific gravity of milk?
Q.5: What do you understand by the terms specific gravity, density and center of gravity/mass? How does the presence of gravitational force affects the human body?
Q.6: Why should the principles of center of gravity be considered before undertaking any strenuous activity.
Q.7: What role does the center of gravity have to play in a normal upright person carrying a large basin of water and a person with crutches, explain?

■ BIBLIOGRAPHY

1. ASBC Methods of Analysis Preface to Table 1: Extract in Wort and Beer, American Society of Brewing Chemists, St Paul, 2009.
2. Dana ES. A Textbook of Mineralogy: With an Extended Treatise on Crystallography. New York, London (Chapman Hall): John Wiley and Sons, 1992.
3. Fox RW, McDonald AT. Introduction to Fluid Mechanics (4th edn). Wiley, 2003.
4. Hough JS, Briggs DE, Stevens R, et al. Malting and Brewing Science, Vol. II, Hopped Wort and Beer, Chapman and Hall, London, 1991.
5. Munson BR, Young DF, Okishi TH. Fundamentals of Fluid Mechanics (4th edn.). Wiley, 2001.
6. Schetz JA, Fuh E. Fundamentals of Fluid Mechanics. Wiley, John and Sons, Incorporated, 1999.
7. Atomi Y. Gravitational Effects on Human Physiology. Subcell Biochem. 2015;72:627-59. doi: 10.1007/978-94-017-9918-8_29. PMID: 26174402.

CHAPTER 4

Force, Energy and Work

Suresh K Sharma, Navjot Kaur

Chapter Outline
- Force
- Newton's Law of Motion
- Forces in the Circular Motion
- Work
- Energy
- Types and Transformation of Energy
- Energy in the Body
- Power
- Principles of Machines
- Efficiency and Mechanical Advantage of a Machine
- Principles of Friction
- Body Mechanics
- Simple Machine
- Lever
- Pulley
- Traction
- Inclined Plane
- Screw
- Application of Principles of gravity in Nursing

■ FORCE

We all have a basic understanding of force from everyday experience. An object (such as a drug trolley) at rest cannot change its position unless it is pushed or pulled. You exert a force on a ball when you throw or kick it. We have to push the drug into the syringe while giving the injection. Similarly, a car or a train moving at a constant speed cannot be stopped unless brakes are applied. In these examples, the word force is associated with muscular activity and some change in the velocity of an object. You should realize that a force is applied through the brakes in a direction opposite to the motion. These examples lead us to define force as:

"Force changes the state of rest or of uniform motion of a body".

There are three defining characteristics of force:
- It starts with an interaction between two or more physical objects (which could include the air)
- The interaction causes a push or pull to occur between the objects
- The resulting push or pull has a direction associated with it

Forces do not always cause motion, however. For example, as you sit reading this book, a gravitational force acts on your body, and yet you are stationary. As a second example, you can push (i.e., exert a force) on a large wall and not be able to move it.

A force produces acceleration in its direction. If several forces are acting on an object, the object accelerates only if the net force acting on it is not zero. Net force or resultant force is the vector sum of all the forces acting on the object. If the net force on a body is zero, then its acceleration will be zero, and it remains either at rest or moving at a constant velocity. A body is said to be in equilibrium when its velocity is constant (zero acceleration) or it is at rest.

So far we have considered only examples where one force was acting on the body, but often several forces act on the same body. Traction is an example of several forces on muscles. When a block is moving on a horizontal surface under the action of some external force, four forces are acting on it: External force (responsible for the motion of the block), the contact force of the surface, frictional, force, and gravitational force of the earth. Similarly, you can easily visualize various forces acting on a flying airplane:
- Force of gravity
- The force of air on the wings and body of the plane
- The force is associated with engine thrust.

■ UNITS OF MEASUREMENT

The SI unit of force is Newton (N). A force of 1N applied to a mass of 1 kilogram produces an acceleration of 1 m/s^2. Force is a vector quantity. To describe a force, we must specify three things its magnitude, its direction, and its point of application.

■ NEWTON'S LAW OF MOTION

Facts related to the motion were first enunciated by Sir Isaac Newton in the form of his famous laws of motion. In 1687, Newton introduced the three laws in his book "Philosophiae Naturalis Principia Mathematica" (Mathematical Principles of Natural Philosophy), which is generally referred to as the "Principia." This is where he also introduced his theory of universal gravitation, thus laying the entire foundation of classical mechanics in one volume.

Newton's First Law

Stated in Newton's words, the first law of motion is:

"Everybody continues in its state of rest or of uniform motion in a straight line unless it is compelled to change that state by forces impressed upon it". This is sometimes called the Law of Inertia, or just inertia. Essentially, it makes the following two points:
- An object that is not moving will not move until a force acts upon it.
- An object that is in motion will not change velocity (or stop) until a force acts upon it.

We come across numerous illustrations of the first law in our daily lives. Some such situations are discussed below:
- Sitting loosely or standing on a bus, we experience a backward jerk when the bus suddenly starts. This is because the lower part of the body moves forward with the bus, whereas the upper part tends to remain at rest.
- While handling the wheelchair, both starting and stopping should be gradual. If the wheelchair suddenly gets into motion, the patient's head may be thrown back, causing an injury. Likewise, if a moving wheelchair is suddenly stopped, the patient may fall forward to the ground.
- A bed at rest has a tendency to stay at rest. We need to apply a large force to move it and when it is set into motion, it continues to be in motion. Force of friction opposes the motion, and so it requires some force (which is less than the force needed to start or stop the motion) to keep it moving. We thus conclude that, due to the inertia of motion, it is easier to keep the bed moving, then to start and stop suddenly.
- You may have seen a person fall on the road while getting down from a moving bus. This is because the lower part of the body comes to rest suddenly, while the upper part tends to continue in a state of motion. So to avoid falls, it is advisable to run for a while with the vehicle.
- Consider a stationary car that is struck from behind by another vehicle. The forces act through the seat, and move the trunk of the driver ahead. But, the inertia of the driver's head causes it to stay in place in the position of rest. Such accidents cause severe stretching of the neck. This can lead to injury of the neck in the cervical region

of the spine. To reduce the impact of the collision, seat belts are provided in automobiles.
- Apart from inertia, another aspect of the first law is force. Since a body cannot change its state of rest or of uniform motion unless an external force acts on it, we can define force with the help of this law as:
- *"Force is an external cause which changes or tends to change the state of rest or the state of uniform motion of a body".*
- A force can change the speed of the body, direction of motion of the body, or shape of the body. That is, force produces acceleration in the body on which it acts. When a force is applied to a stationary body, it starts moving. Its initial velocity was zero; the force produced acceleration in the body, making it move faster.

Newton's Second Law

Imagine performing an experiment in which you push a book across a frictionless table. When you exert some horizontal force 'F' on the book, it moves with some acceleration 'a'. If you apply a force twice as great, you find that the acceleration of the book doubles. If you increase the applied force to 3F, the acceleration triples, and so on.

From such observations, we conclude that the acceleration of an object is directly proportional to the force acting on it.

The acceleration of an object also depends on its mass, as stated in the preceding section. We can understand this from the previous thought experiment. If you apply a force 'F' to a book on a frictionless table, the book undergoes some acceleration 'a'. If the mass of the book is doubled, the same applied force produces acceleration $a/2$. If the mass is tripled, the same applied force produces acceleration $a/3$.

If you are struck by a fast-moving cricket ball, you get injured. However, a flower moving with same velocity as of cricket ball and hit you, it will not cause injury or pain. Similarly, if the ball is moving slowly, the injury will be less serious. This suggests that an impact made by an object depends on two things: it's mass and velocity. So, Newton felt the necessity of defining a quantity called linear momentum (p) as the product of mass and velocity. Mathematically, we can write

$$p = mv$$

Linear momentum, 'p' is a vector quantity in the direction of velocity. The above equation mathematically can be restated as follows:

$$F = ma$$

where 'F' is the net force acting on the body, 'm' is its mass, and 'a' is the acceleration in the direction of the net force.

According to Newton, the second law of motion is:

"The magnitude of the resultant force acting on a body is proportional to the product of the mass of the body and its acceleration. The direction of the force is the same as that of the acceleration".

The acceleration produced in a body by a force depends on the mass of the body. For example, if the same force is applied to two beds one empty and another with a patient, the empty bed is lighter and moves faster than a loaded bed. In other words, if equal forces are applied to two objects; one with a smaller mass and another larger mass, more acceleration is acquired by an object having a smaller mass. A larger force must be applied to the loaded bed for it to have the same acceleration.

So, Newton's first law of motion enables us to define inertia and the second law gives us a quantitative measure of force. In simple words, Newton's first law explains what happens to an object when no forces act on it. It either remains at rest or moves in a straight line with constant speed. Newton's second law answers the question of what happens to an object that has a nonzero resultant force acting on it.

You now know that forces cause a change in the motion of a body. But how do we exert a force on this body? Inevitably, there is an agent who makes it possible. Very often, your feet (while playing football) or hands (while playing volleyball) are the agents. That is, forces arise from interactions between systems. This information is contained in the third law of motion.

Newton's Third Law

Stated in Newton's words, the third law of motion is as follows:

"To every action, there is always an equal and opposite reaction".

An important consequence of this law is that forces always appear in pairs; a single isolated force never exists. The action and reaction forces act on different objects and must be of the same type.

If two objects interact, the force F_{12} exerted by object 1 on object 2 is equal in magnitude and opposite in direction to the force F_{21} exerted by object 2 on object 1:

$$F_{12} = F_{21}$$

Remember, the two forces in an action-reaction pair always act on two different objects.

To elaborate on the third law of motion, let us consider a book kept on a table. The book exerts a force, equal to its weight, on the table. But if this were the only force, the book would have gone through the table. Since it does not happen, the motion of the book (due to the force of its own weight) must have been resisted by an equal and opposite force exerted on it in the upward direction by the table.

Similarly, the weight of the body of a patient lying in bed pushes against the mattress. In turn, the mattress pushes him upwards. The third law helps us understand why patients in bed for a long period of time, develop bedsores. This is because the heavier parts of the body (bony parts) press more firmly against the mattress than do the lighter portions and, in turn, receive a greater reaction force. The reaction force interferes with the normal circulation of blood to the tissues and causes pressure sores.

Frictional Force

Frictional force refers to the force generated by two surfaces that contact and slide against each other. These forces are mainly affected by the surface texture and quantity of force requiring them together. The angle and position of the object affect the volume of frictional force. When an object is in motion either on a surface or in a viscous medium such as water or air, there is resistance to motion because the object interacts with its surroundings. This resistance is called the force of friction. If an object is placed against an object, then the frictional force will be the same as the weight of the object. If an object is pushed against the surface, then the frictional force will be increased and become extra than the weight of the object. The friction force is an important part of our day-to-day life activities. We cannot move, if there were no friction. However, it is undesirable in machines.

Experiments show that the friction forces come into existence from the nature of the two surfaces, because of their roughness, contact is made only at a few points of the surface where peaks of the material. The detailed analysis of friction is quite complex at the atomic level, frictional force ultimately involves an electrical interaction between atoms or molecules.

To move joints in our body, we have to overcome friction. If frictional forces become large, some diseases of joints develop. Similarly, friction can cause bedsores in a patient, particularly when he/ she is confined to bed for a long period. The synovial fluid in the joints acts as a lubricant which reduces frictional force. Similarly, saliva lubricates the mouth. Most of the large organs in the human body are in constant motion. The heart, lungs, and intestines have a rhythmic motion. In all these organs, a slippery mucous covering minimizes the friction. Further, while inserting gastric tubes, rectal tubes, and catheter, you might have used one or the other lubricant to minimize irritation of the membranes inside the body caused due to friction.

■ PRINCIPLES OF FRICTION

- ❖ Friction is the force that opposes the movement of one body over the surface of another body. The heat produced by friction is known as internal energy. Friction may be both advantageous and disadvantageous depending on the desired therapeutic effect.
- ❖ When two solid objects, slip over each other, the frictional force is called kinetic friction. When two objects do not slip over each other, the frictional force is called static friction.
- ❖ In hospitals and nursing homes, a useful safety measure is to block off areas of flooring being scrubbed and dry the floors carefully before they are walked on.
- ❖ Friction is necessary for striking a matching effect. Without friction, screws and nails would not hold wood together. Rubber tips at the bottom of crutches provide sufficient friction to keep the crutches from slipping.
- ❖ Friction may sometimes be disadvantageous. Rubber tubes such as gastric and duodenal tubes, catheters, and renal tubes may irritate the membranes over which they pass unless measures are taken to prevent friction. Therefore, the lubricant is used to minimize friction.
- ❖ Medication in tablet or capsule form is generally administered with water to prevent friction between the outer surface of the medication and the tissues of the mouth and throat.
- ❖ Frictional forces are reduced by serous fluids wherever motion occurs in the body. For example, synovial fluid in the joints and the serous fluid between the layers of the pleura, pericardium, and peritoneum.

Fluid friction is a term applied to the friction of solids passing through fluids such as the blood cells through the blood.

Gravitational Force

Another very common force is the gravitational force, which the earth exerts on all bodies. The gravitational force is a force that attracts any two objects with mass. We call the gravitational force attractive because it always tries to pull masses together, it never pushes them apart. In fact, every object, including us, is pulling on every other object in the entire universe. This is called Newton's universal law of gravitation. In fact, the weight of a body is actually the force of gravitational attraction between the body and the earth. During a blood transfusion, blood gets from the hanging bag to the patient's body because of the gravitational force. The gravitational force on the skeleton contributes to healthy bones.

■ FORCES IN THE CIRCULAR MOTION

Uniform Circular Motion

The movement of a body following a circular path is called a circular motion. Now, the motion of a body moving with constant speed along a circular path is called uniform circular motion. Here, the speed is constant, but the velocity changes. You know that no force acts on a body (along the direction of motion) moving with uniform velocity along a straight line. Now consider the motion of a planet around the sun. The planet Jupiter, 300 times more massive than Earth, circles the sun at a speed of 13 km per second. Similarly, we may imagine the rotation of wheels in machinery or a merry-go-round. These are examples of circular motion. The question is: What happens to the direction of motion in such cases? The direction of motion of a body in circular motion changes continuously. Thus, a body in uniform circular motion has the variable velocity as direction is changing continuously. In other words, uniform circular motion is an example of accelerated motion. Mainly there are two forces namely centripetal and centrifugal forces, which give rise to circular motion, as detailed below:

Centripetal Force

When an object is moving in a circular path with constant speed, a constant force acts on the object. This force acts along a direction perpendicular to the direction of motion. (This is because any component in the direction of motion would also produce a change in the speed of the object and the motion will not be uniform).

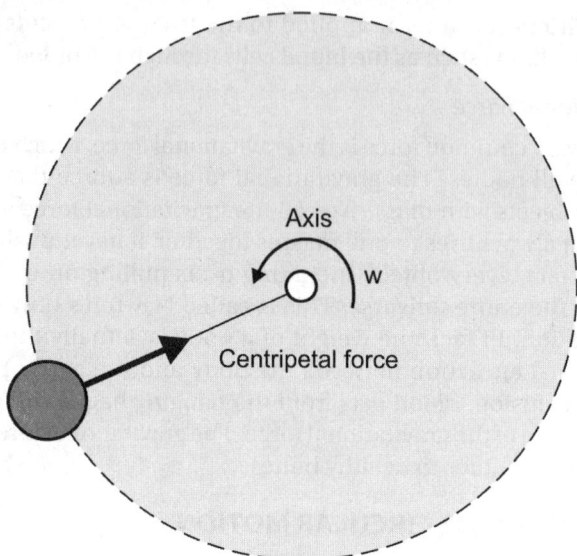

Fig. 4.1: Centripetal force.

The force responsible for the constant acceleration directed towards the center of the circle is called the centripetal force **(Fig. 4.1)**. You may recall playing with a top (lattu). You must have seen a cyclist turning a corner. He inclines his body towards the center of the curved path. By doing this, he gets the required centripetal force and ensures safety around a curve. Similarly, a racing track for motor cars is constructed in such a way that it banks inwards and provides the centripetal force.

Centrifugal Force

Tie a stone to a piece of a string and move it along a circular path around your hand. The stone moves with a constant speed along a circle. Velocity is changing because of the direction of motion is changing continuously. Hence, it is accelerated motion. Thus, a force must be acting on it. This is the force of the string pulling the stone inward. It is called the centripetal force.

Now, according to Newton's third law of motion, for every action on one body, there arises a force of reaction which is equal in magnitude but opposite in direction. In the case of uniform circular motion, a centripetal force acts on the revolving body (stone) and is directed towards the center. An equal and opposite force of reaction keeps the stone from falling inwards. This force is directed away from the center and is known as centrifugal force. If the string breaks, there

CHAPTER 4: Force, Energy and Work

will be no centripetal or centrifugal force acting on the stone or the hand respectively, and the stone would follow a straight-line path, which is tangent to the circle at the instant of time.

The centripetal force causes a body to move in a circular path of the constant radius by constantly pulling it toward the center which it describes. Since the speed is constant, this force changes only the direction of motion. The body pulls outward against this change in motion with a force called centrifugal force **(Fig. 4.2)**.

You come across a variety of situations or must have seen a variety of machines which involves circular motion and the concept of centripetal and centrifugal forces. We discuss some of them in the following:

❖ In the laundry, wet laundry is dried by spinning the cylinders at high speeds, which causes the drops of water to fly in front.
❖ In a circus, motorcyclist in death well makes use of centrifugal force to avoid fall.
❖ When a nurse shakes down a thermometer in a circular path, she causes the heaving substance mercury to be thrown, to the bottom.
❖ In a chemical lab, a centrifuge is used to separate chemicals in a solution. An ultracentrifuge enables us to determine the molecular weight of large macromolecules.

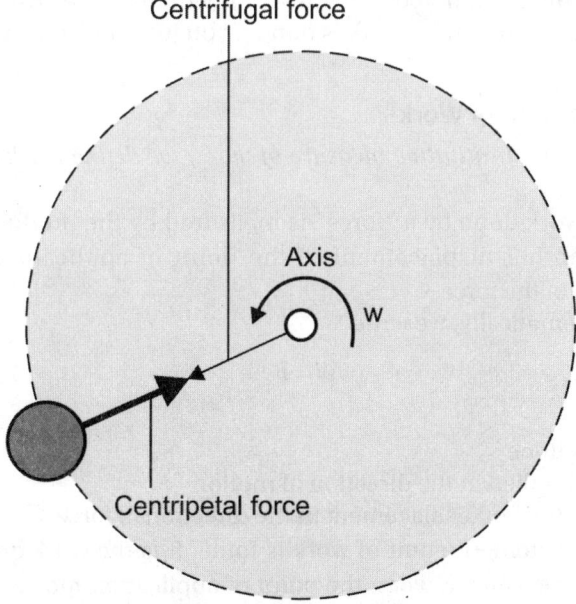

Fig. 4.2: Centrifugal force.

❖ Further, you know that blood is a mixture of particles (cells, protein molecules, water molecules, etc.) of various weights and sizes. If a blood sample is placed in a centrifuge and rotated at high speeds, it separates into layers containing particles of different densities. The particles of maximum density form a layer in the bottom of the test tube (outer region of the circular path) whereas those of minimum density moves towards the top (the mouth of the tube).

■ WORK

When a force acts upon an object to cause a displacement of the object, it is said that work was done upon the object. There are three key ingredients to workforce, displacement, and cause. In order for a force to qualify as having done work on an object, there must be a displacement and the force must cause the displacement. In other words, work is done by a force when its point of application moves in the direction of the force. When the point of application moves against the direction of the force, work is said to be done against the force. For example, a nurse lifting a baby from the crib does some work against gravity. Similarly, work is done in shifting a patient from bed to trolley or wheelchair. Even while giving intramuscular (IM) or intravenous (IV) injection, work is done on the piston of the syringe. An important point to note here, from a physics point of view, if the point of application does not move, no work is done. Thus, in the language of physics, no work is done if you just hold a baby in your arms.

Measurement of Work

To obtain a quantitative measure of work, we define work done as follows:

The work done by a "force" is measured by the product of the force, another displacement of the point of application in the direction of the force.

Mathematically, we write

$$W = F \cdot d$$

where,
W = work done
F = force applied in the direction of motion
d = magnitude of displacement in the direction of force

In SI system, the unit of work is Joule. It is the work done by a force of one Newton when the point of application moves through one meter in the direction of the force.

$$1 J = 1 N \times 1 m$$

A smaller unit of work is 'erg' which is the work done by a force of one dyne when the body moves through a distance of one cm. The relation between Joule and erg is:

$$1 J = 10^7 \text{ erg}$$

Work is done when a person climbs a hill or walks upstairs. It is equal to the product of a person's weight (mg) and the vertical distance (h) moved. You may ask: Is work done when a person is running on a leveled smooth surface at constant speed? In the language of physics, no work is done because weight is acting along a direction normal to his motion. However, his muscles are doing (internal) work; which appears as heat and raises his body temperature. The heat generated due, to this internal work is removed from the body by the blood flow, condition of the skin, and sweating.

■ ENERGY

It is our common experience that we need energy in one form or the other to do work. You know that petrol burnt in a car makes the car move. A raised hammer drives a nail into the wall. A rushing stream can make a wheel rotate. In these examples, the petrol in a car, a raised hammer, and the rushing stream has the ability to work. Thus, an operational definition of energy is:

"The capacity to do work is known as energy".

Our body gets energy from the food we eat. Food energy is used by the body to operate its various organs. Some food energy is also used in maintaining constant body temperature and some part (5%) of food energy is excreted. The remaining energy is retained as fat.

Since the energy content of a body is measured by the total amount of work it can do, the units of work and energy are the same, i.e. energy is also measured in joule (J). In nursing, we use kilocalories to measure food, energy and kilocalories per minute for the rate of heat production. The energy value of food referred to by nutritionists as a calorie is actually a kilocalorie. For example, a diet of 2000 calories per day is 2000 K cal/day.

- ❖ ***Calorie:*** One calorie is defined as the energy required to raise the temperature of one gram of water by 1°C.
- ❖ ***Kilogram Calorie:*** It is the large calorie used in nutrition and the amount of heat required to raise the temperature of 1000 cc (1 liter) of water to 1°C. It is abbreviated by K cal.

❖ **Kilowatt-hour (kWh):** It is a unit to measure electrical energy. 1 kWh is equal to energy consumed by 1 kW power device in one hour.
  • All these units of energy or energy consumed are related to each other. The conversion factors are given in **Table 4.1**.

Table 4.1: Energy conversion factor.

Unit	Joule (J)	Kilowatt-hour (kWh)	Calories (cal)
1 J	1	2.78×10^{-7}	0.239
1 Cal	4.186	1.16×10^{-6}	1
1 kWh	3.6×10^6	1	8.6×10^5

■ TYPES AND TRANSFORMATION OF ENERGY

In nature, energy exists in various different forms. Depending on its source, energy can be classified as mechanical, heat, sound, light, electrical, magnetic, chemical or nuclear. Physics in many ways is the study of energy in its various forms. But here we shall confine ourselves to different forms of energy in the body and its conversion from one form to another. For instance, chemical energy in the body is converted into mechanical work and used up in other life-preserving functions.

Kinetic Energy: It is the energy associated with motion. The kinetic energy (KE) of a moving object is calculated by:
$$KE = \frac{1}{2} mv^2$$
Here, m = mass of object and v = velocity.

Potential Energy: Potential energy is present in the universe in many forms, including gravitational, electromagnetic, chemical, and nuclear. It is stored energy and depends on an object's position or composition. The stored energy is potential energy because it is potentially available to be changed to kinetic energy **(Fig. 4.3)**. For example, in an electric motor connected to a battery, the chemical energy in the battery is converted to kinetic energy as the shaft of the motor turns. The transformation of energy from one form to another is an essential part of the study of physics, engineering, chemistry, biology, geology, and astronomy.

For gravitational systems,
$$PE = wh$$
where,
w = weight
h = height

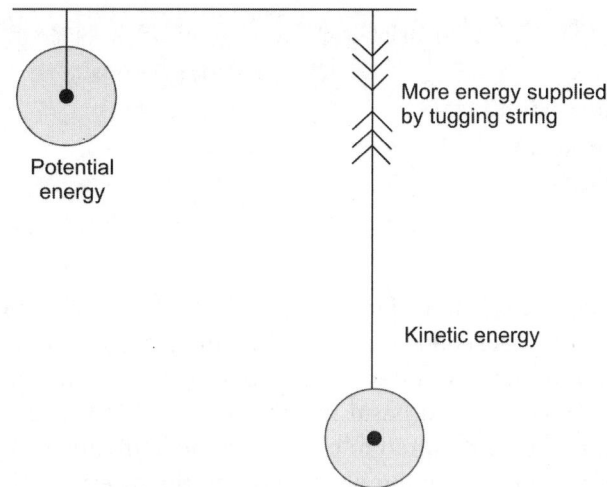

Fig. 4.3: Potential and kinetic energy

Example: When the left ventricle forces blood into the aorta, the aorta expands and stores potential energy by virtue of the work done upon it in producing the expansion. When aorta relaxes, the potential energy is changed to kinetic energy, which aids in pushing the blood through the aorta to other arteries.

■ ENERGY IN THE BODY

Energy is a primary importance for our body. Our body requires energy for its various activities. Even while resting, about one fourth of the body energy is used by the muscles and the heart. Even in rest, body energy is used by the brain, kidneys, liver, and spleen. While working, apart from providing energy to various organs, body energy is utilized in maintaining a constant body temperature. Some parts of the body energy is excreted. If the intake of energy is more, the unused part is stored as body fat. It is for this reason that, to get rid of unnecessary body fat, doctors advise regular exercise to persons not undertaking much physical work. The basic source of body energy is the food we eat. You must realize that the food is not used directly in the form of energy. Our body converts this food into energy.

Thus, the human body derives its energy from food. This energy is released as energy for metabolism when food is oxidized in the cells of the body. The rate of oxidation is called the metabolic rate.

The caloric values of some types of food converted into energy due to oxidation are given in **Table 4.2**. These are the maximum expected values. In actual practice, all this energy is not available.

Table 4.2: Typical energy values of selected food types.

Food	Calorie value (kcal g−1)
Glucose	3.8
Carbohydrate	4.1
Proteins	4.1
Fats	9.3

This is because the oxidation may not be complete. The unutilized products are released in feces, urine, and intestinal gas.

A normal person under resting conditions requires nearly 92 kcal/hr. This so-called basal metabolic rate (BMR) signifies the minimum energy required to perform basic body functions (such as breathing and pumping blood through the arteries). The BMR primarily depends upon thyroid function, an overactive thyroid has a higher BMR. The BMR of a living being is proportional to its mass.

Suppose you are required to advise people to reduce weight or keep a constant weight. An individuals desirous of keeping a constant weight should consume just enough food to provide for BMR plus physical activities. Eating too little causes weight loss. And if continued for long, it results in starvation. However, a diet in excess of the requirements of the body causes an increase in weight. To lose weight, we should be careful about the quantity of food we eat and avoid fat-rich foods. This is because the caloric value of fats is almost twice the value of proteins or carbohydrates.

■ CONSERVATION OF ENERGY

You now know that our body gets energy from food in the form of chemical energy. The chemical energy stored in our body, in turn, changes into mechanical energy (external work, breathing, pumping blood), and electrical energy (control of muscles and organ responses). We, therefore, find that the transformation of energy from one form to another takes place in almost every physical activity. But energy is indestructible. That is, energy is never destroyed; it simply changes its form. In other words, energy is conserved. This constitutes the law governing the conservation of energy:

"Energy can neither be created nor destroyed. It can change from one form to another; the total amount of energy remains unchanged."

This is one of the most fundamental principles of science. The conservation of energy in the body can be expressed as:

Change in stored energy in the body = Heat lost from the body + Work done

Here we have assumed that no food or drink is taken in and no feces or urine is excreted during the time considered.

■ POWER

We have not yet talked about the time interval during which a task or work is done. We can define power as the rate of doing work, it is the work done in unit time. Because work is energy transfer, power is also the rate at which energy is expended. If an external force 'F' is applied to an object and work done by this force in time interval 't' is 'W', then average power during this interval is defined as:

$$P = \frac{W}{t}$$

The SI unit of power is Joules per second (J/s), also called the watt (W) (after James Watt). Another common unit of power is horsepower (hp). 1 hp is equal to 746 watt.

■ PRINCIPLES OF MACHINES

Mechanics is a branch of physics. In general, mechanics allows one to describe and predict the conditions of rest or movement of particles and bodies subjected to the action of forces. Aristotle was among the first scholars to introduce the term mechanics.

- ❖ *Simple Machines:* Machines are devices for transferring energy or transforming energy into work. Machines operate by receiving mechanical, heat, electrical, chemical, or other forms of energy, and by doing work they transfer the energy to the body upon which the work is done. For example, when a nurse injects a hypodermic medication, energy is transferred from the nurse's muscles to the syringe and needle. The muscles of the body are examples of machines that transform potential energy stored in chemicals in the muscles into kinetic energy of motion.
- ❖ Simple machines help us to get work done more easily. Usually, a simple machine helps to overcome a force applied at some point of it by means of another force applied at some other convenient point. The applied force invariably differs in magnitude or direction or both. The force that is overcome by the machine is called 'load'. It is usually the weight of a body to be lifted. The applied force to overcome the load is called the 'effort'.
- ❖ *Principles:* When work is done by the machine, the resistance (R) moves through a distance (dr). When work is done on the machine, the effort (E) also acts through a distance (de).

❖ Theoretically, in an ideal machine

$$\text{Input} = \text{Output}$$
$$\text{Or}$$
$$E \times de = R \times dr$$

■ EFFICIENCY AND MECHANICAL ADVANTAGE OF A MACHINE

The efficiency of a machine is the ratio of its output work to its input work expressed in percent, i.e.,

$$\text{Efficiency} = \frac{\text{Work output}}{\text{Work input}} \times 10$$

The mechanical advantage (MA) of a machine is the ratio of the resistance to the effort, i.e.,

$$MA = \frac{R}{L}$$

Mechanical advantage may also be obtained by the ratio of the distance through which the effort acts to the distance, through which the resistance moves, i.e.,

$$MA = \frac{dr}{de}$$

■ BODY MECHANICS

The efficiency of the human body as a machine is obtained by using the relation:

$$\text{Efficiency} = \frac{\text{Work done}}{\text{Energy consumed}}$$

The efficiency of man for some activities is given in **Table 4.3**. You will note that the values are much less than 100%. One of the major reasons for the low efficiency of human beings is the presence of friction between joints. To minimize friction, the human body has an inherent mechanism of lubrication. The saliva we add when we chew food acts as a lubricant. Similarly, the heart, lungs, and intestines are lubricated by a slippery mucus covering.

Table 4.3: Mechanical efficiency of human beings.

Table	Efficiency (%)
Cycling	~20
Swimming	<2
Shoveling	~3

Body mechanics is a term used to describe the ways we move as we go about our daily lives. It includes how we hold our bodies when we sit, stand, lift, carry, bend, and sleep.

Principles of Body Mechanics
- The wider the base of support, the greater the stability of the body.
- The lower the center of gravity, the greater the stability of the body.
- The equilibrium of an object is maintained as long as the line of gravity passes through its base of support.
- Facing the direction of movement prevents abnormal twisting of the spine.
- Dividing balanced activity between arms and legs reduces the risk of back injury.
- Maintaining good body mechanics reduces fatigue of the muscle groups.

■ LEVER

A lever is an example of a simple machine. It is a rigid bar that moves about a fixed axis called the fulcrum (f). The bar may be straight or bent. In addition to a fulcrum, the lever consists of two forces:
- Effort (E)
- Resistance (R)

The machine law describes the relationship between the load lifted (W) and the effort applied (P).

$$P = mW + C$$

Where,
P = Effort applied
W = Load lifted
m = Constant equal to the slope of the line
C = Exhibits mechanical friction

Holds true for all levers in the friction is neglected. Like any simple machine, a force FE is applied on one end of the bar and a load force FL is balanced. The mechanical advantage (MA) of the lever is defined as:

$$MA = \frac{FL}{EF}$$

If the MA is greater than 1, the machine helps us do work more easily. Depending upon the relative positions of the load, effort, and fulcrum, levers are classified into three classes:
1. **First class levers:** In this class of lever, the fulcrum is situated somewhere in between the effort and the resistance **(Fig. 4.4)**. Scissors, and hemostats are examples of such a machine. In the

human body, a first-class lever is represented by the triceps and brachial muscles.

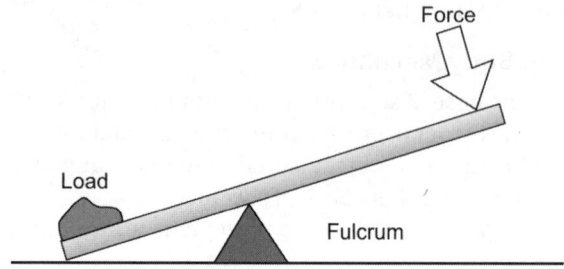

Fig. 4.4: First class lever.

2. **Second class levers:** In this class of lever, the resistance is situated between the fulcrum and the effort **(Fig. 4.5)**. Wheelbarrow and oxygen cylinder carrier are examples of second class levers.

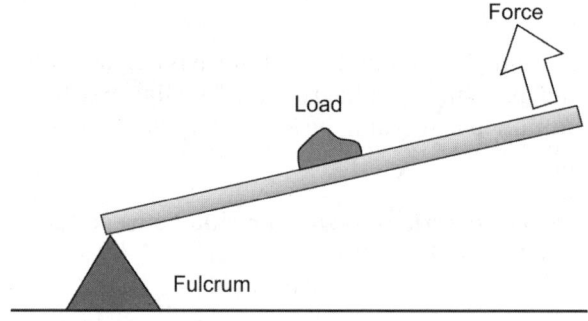

Fig. 4.5: Second class lever.

3. **Third class levers:** In a third class lever, the effort is situated between the resistance and the fulcrum **(Fig. 4.6)**. Forceps and the action of the biceps brachii are the examples of third class lever.

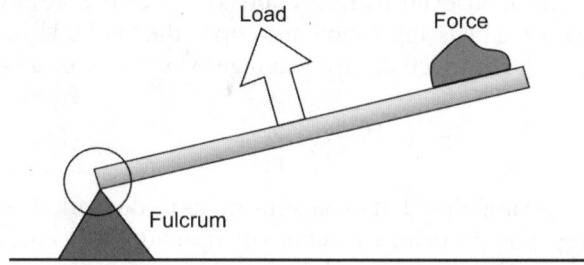

Fig. 4.6: Third class lever.

The Class III levers are most common in the human body. Class II levers are next and Class I levers are the least common.

In an automobile, the force of the engine is transformed into another suitable force that rotates the wheels and makes the vehicle move.

The work done on the machine is the product of the effort and the distance through which the effort to act. The work done by the machine is the product of the load and the distance through which the output force acts. Theoretically, in an ideal machine, we expect that the work done on the machine will be equal to the work done by the machine.

■ LEVER ACTION OF JAW

The upper jaw maxilla is a fixed frame. The lower jaw mandible is movable about a fulcrum S within the skull. The effort tension E is applied by the masseter muscles situated on, both sides of the face. When we bite something using our front-cutting teeth incisors, we try to overcome the load W_1 situated between our teeth. The system acts as a Class III lever. However, when we crack a nut or chew something with deeper molars, the system is transformed into a Class II lever with muscle effort acting over the load W_2 **(Fig. 4.7)**.

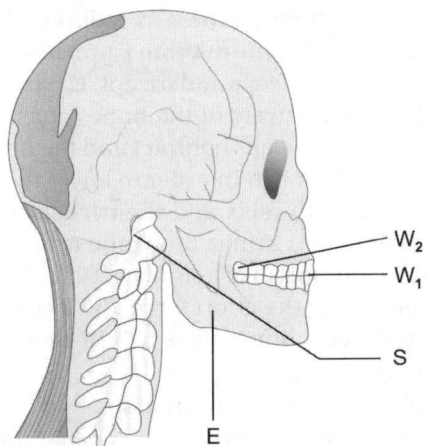

Fig. 4.7: Lever action of jaw.

■ LEVER ACTION OF FOOT

When a person stands on one foot and raises his heels, a reaction force W equals the weight of the body, acts upwards at the midpoint between ball B and ankle joint of the foot. The effort required to raise the heel is applied on the heel bone as an upward pull P via tissues known as the Achilles tendon. The system may be considered equivalent, to a Class II lever with the fulcrum situated at the ball of the foot **(Fig. 4.8)**.

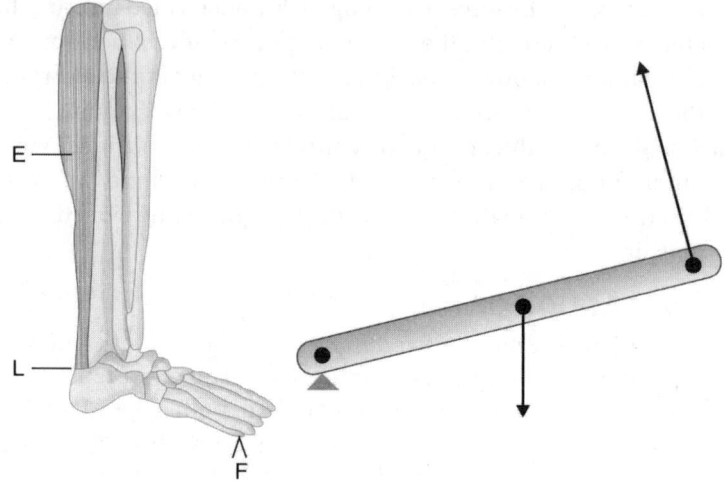

Fig. 4.8: Lever action of foot.

■ LEVER ACTION OF FOREARM

When we lift a load W bones known as radius and ulna constitute the lever arm BC, pivoted at the fulcrum F provided by another bone humerus. Muscles called biceps and triceps, can exert tension forces at points A and C, respectively of the bones constituting the lever BC. When we lift a load, biceps contract and the arm flexes. During this action, triceps do not act. In order to lower the raised forearm, the biceps are allowed to relax and the triceps come into action. The resulting lever action brings down the arm. When the biceps provides the effort, our forearm acts like a Class III lever and when the triceps are providing the effort force, the forearm forms a Class I lever. Note that the arm bones have two-in-one lever mechanism of action **(Fig. 4.9)**.

They all apply forces by means of levers that have a mechanical advantage. But this arrangement provides greater speed to the limbs. A small change in the length of the muscle produces a relatively larger displacement of the limb's extremities. It seems that nature prefers speed to strength. In fact, the speeds attainable at limb extremities are remarkable. A skilled person can throw a stone at a speed in excess of 100 mph. Which was useful for survival in Stone Age.

Liver Action at Hip Joint

The hip joint for a male and its simplified lever representation, giving dimensions are stabilized in its socket by a group of muscles,

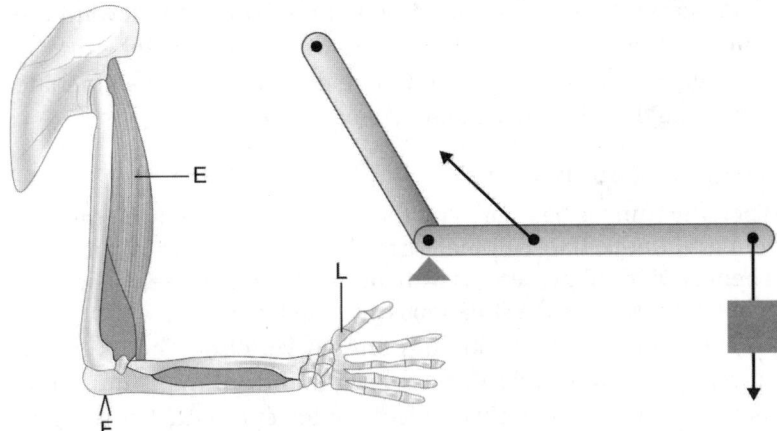

Fig. 4.9: Lever action of forearm.

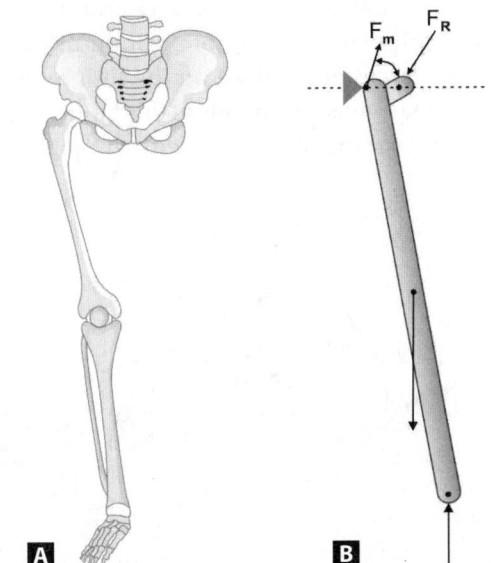

Figs. 10.10A and B: (A) The hip; (B) Its lever representation.

represented in **Figs. 10.10A and B** as a single resultant force F_m, WL represents the combined weight of the leg, foot, and thigh. Typically, this weight is a fraction (0.185) of the total body weight (W). The weight WL is assumed to act vertically downward at the midpoint of the limb. The force on the hip joint is nearly two and one-half times the weight of the person.

Persons who have an injured hip, limp by leaning toward the injured side as they step on that foot. As a result, the center of gravity of the body shifts into a position more directly above the hip joint, decreasing the force on the injured area.

Liver Action at the Back

When the trunk is bent forward, the spine pivots mainly on the fifth lumbar vertebra. If we will analyze the forces involved when the trunk is bent at 60° from the vertical with the arms hanging freely. The lever model representing the situation is given in **Fig. 4.11**.

The pivot point A is the fifth lumbar vertebra. The lever arm AB represents the back. The weight of the trunk W_1 is uniformly distributed along the back; its effect can be represented by a weight suspended in the middle. The weight of the head and arms is represented by W_2 suspended at the end of the lever arm. The erector spinalis muscle, shown as the connection D-C attached at a point two-thirds up the spine, maintains the position of the back. This indicates that large forces are exerted on the fifth lumbar vertebra and backaches originate most frequently at this point. So the position shown in the figure is not the recommended way of lifting a weight.

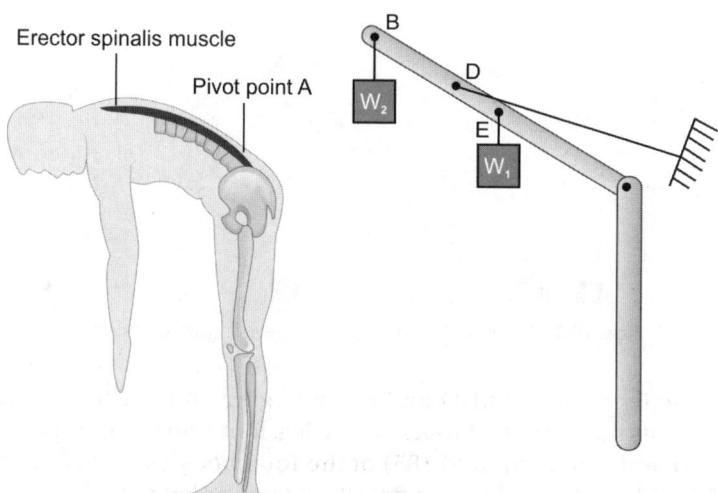

Fig. 4.11: The bent back (Left). Lever representation (Right).

■ PULLEY

A pulley consists of a wheel without a grooved rim around which a string can be passed. The pulley rotates about an axel through its center. The axle is supported by a framework called a block **(Fig. 4.12)**.

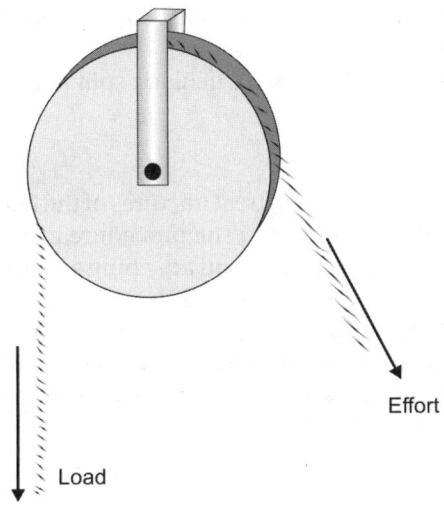

Fig. 4.12: Pulley.

Pulleys are classified as:
- *Fixed pulleys:* They are attached to some fixed support.
- *Movable pulleys:* They are attached to the resistance and move along with the resistance.

The chief function of the pulley wheel is to equalize the tension of the string on either side of it.

■ TRACTION

Traction can be used to realign a fractured bone or other dislocated body part. It uses weights, pulleys, and ropes to apply gentle pressure and pull the injured or broken part back into place. Three types of traction are there mainly: skin traction, skeletal traction, and cervical traction. The type of traction required will depend on the severity and location of the injury or broken bone.

The Purpose of Traction

Traction is used to stabilize fractures or injuries and to restore tension to surrounding tissues, muscles, tendons, and other structures. Traction can be used to:
- Stabilize and realign broken bones or dislocated parts of the body

(such as the shoulder).
- Restore the bone's normal position after it has been broken.
- To reduce the pressure on the spine, stretch the neck and realign the vertebrae.
- Temporarily reduce pain before surgery.
- Reduce or eliminate muscle spasms, constricted joints, muscles, and tendonitis.
- Reduce pressure on nerves, particularly spinal nerves.
- Treat bone deformities.

Skeletal Traction

Skeletal traction can be used to treat fractures of the femur, pelvis, hip, and certain upper arm fractures. The procedure involves inserting a wire or pin directly into the bone and attaching weights using pulleys or ropes that regulate the pressure. Skeletal traction can be used to treat fractures that are more severe than others. It allows for greater weight to be added to the bone with less chance of damaging the soft tissues. Skeletal traction is performed under anesthesia to ensure that patient does not feel any pain.

Skin Traction

Skin traction is less intrusive than skeletal traction. It uses splints and bandages on the area of the fracture. The adhesive tapes are then applied to the skin. Pressure is applied by attaching weights and pulleys. The muscles and tendons pull an extremity to a shorter or bent position when a bone is broken. The traction can help to hold the fractured bone and dislocated joints in place. This can lead to painful movement and cramping at the fracture site. Buck›s traction, a form of skin traction, is used widely for hip, acetabular, and femoral fractures.

Cervical Traction

When the neck vertebrae have been fractured, cervical traction is used. This type of traction uses a device that circles the head and attaches itself to a harness that wraps around the torso. This stretch to the neck relieves pressure on the spine and aligns the vertebrae.

Risks and Contraindications

Traction poses no risk in the long-term. However, some people might experience pain or muscle spasms in the area being treated.

There are potential dangers associated with traction:
- Negative reactions to anesthesia.
- An excessive amount of bleeding at the location of a pin/screw in skeletal traction.

- Infection at the place where the screw or pin has been inserted.
- Extreme swelling can cause nerve or vascular injuries.
- In cases of skin crackle, there is damage to the surrounding tissue and skin.

Contraindications

Skin traction is not recommended for seniors as their skin may be damaged by the force of the traction. If the patient has any of the following conditions, traction may be contraindicated:
- Osteoporosis
- Rheumatoid arthritis
- Infection
- Pregnancy
- Circulatory and respiratory problems
- Claustrophobia
- Cardiovascular disease
- Joint problems

Before applying, both skin and skeletal tensions require X-rays. To ensure the correct alignment of the bones, these may be repeated throughout the treatment. The severity, location, and extent of injury or broken bone will determine how long the traction will be. The time taken to traction can range from 24 hours up to six weeks or more. Skin traction can be used temporarily to immobilize the fracture while waiting for corrective surgery.

There are many potential problems associated with prolonged immobility in traction such as bedsores also with respiratory, urinary, and circulatory problems. Various physical therapies are recommended to maintain joint and muscle movement. Regular inspections of the equipment will ensure that it is properly positioned and calibrated.

Traction can be a very challenging treatment-physically, emotionally, and psychologically, so as nursing person, we should explain and assist the person and family to cope with this challenging time.

According to balancing forces, we can also classify the tractions as follows:
- **Fixed traction:** In this, a splint such as Thomas splint is employed. In this traction the forward pull of the force (wt) is made directly on the splint **(Fig. 4.13)**.

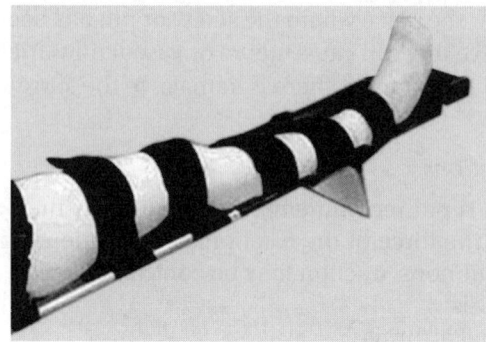

Fig. 4.13: Thomas splint traction.

- ❖ **Balanced traction:** In this, a force is transmitted over a pulley by a cord from a weight hung at the foot, head, or side of the bed. It may be fixed to the injured part by adhesive strapping or by a pin passed directly through the bone **(Fig. 4.14)**.

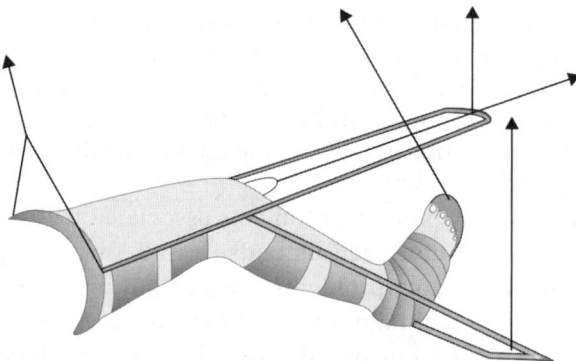

Fig. 4.14: Balanced traction.

- ❖ **Russell traction:** It employs the principle of balanced traction for treating fractures of the femur. In this traction force is applied to a sling placed under the knee. This force is transmitted by a rope, which passes over a pulley to the foot of the bed. Bypassing this rope over another pulley connected to a wooden block and in the adhesive strapping below the patient's foot, the same force is applied to the lower leg **(Fig. 4.15)**.
    - Russell traction is based on the concept of vector addition and equilibrium of forces. The backward pull of the muscles and the counterforce of the patient weight balance the resultant force and keep the fractured ends of the bone in alignment.

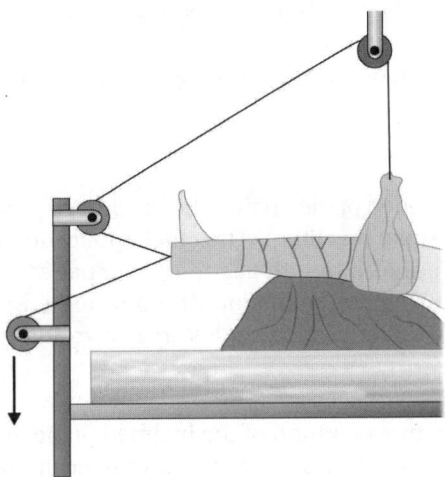

Fig. 4.15: Russell traction.

■ INCLINED PLANE

A ramp used in buildings to join floors of different levels is a practical example of a machine called an inclined plane. It is much easier to wheel a patient up a ramp (the length of the plane) than to raise him bodily from one level to the other (the height of the plane). An inclined plane can handle jobs that we might find dangerous to carry-out **(Fig. 4.16)**.

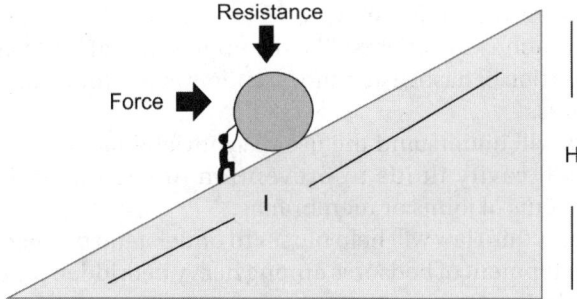

Fig. 4.16: Inclined plane.

The effort (E) is the force parallel to the length of the plane necessary to move the patient and the chair. The distance the effort moves is the length of the inclined plane (l); the distance the resistance (R) is moved vertically is the height of the plane or the distance between the two floor levels (h). The law of the inclined plane is expressed as follows:

$$\text{Effort} \times \text{Length of incline} = \text{Resistance} \times \text{Height of incline}$$
$$El = Rh$$

■ WEDGE

It is a modified inclined plane. In this, the machine is pushed between two objects and separates them. The chief application of the wedge in nursing is its use as a mouth gag to open a patient's mouth after anesthesia or during a convulsion. The beveled edges of chisels, cutting tools, and hypodermic needles are also examples of wedges.

■ SCREW

The screw is also an adaptation of the inclined plane. In a sense, it is like an inclined plane that is wrapped around a cylinder. The screw is used wherever a large resistance is to be overcome by a relatively small effort. For example, jackscrew is used to lift a heavy automobile or truck. There are many pieces of equipment in the hospital that operate on the principle of screw, e.g. crank of a gatch bed, wheel of operating room tables, wheel of an autoclave door. Most common application clinically is that of the crew of a clamp used on rubber tubing. A small effort on the screw produces a large to occlude or lessen the opening of the tube.

■ APPLICATION OF PRINCIPLES OF GRAVITY IN NURSING

- ❖ Knowledge of the friction will help nurses to plan nursing procedures in a manner, where they can minimize the friction and irritations to patients; like the application of lubricating jelly for insertion of nasogastric tubes, endotracheal tubes, and urinary catheters.
- ❖ Nurses will understand the use of synovial fluid or other normal minimal cavity fluids to prevention of friction and smooth movements of joints or membranes.
- ❖ Newton's third law will help nurses to understand the mechanisms of development of bedsores among heavy bedridden patients and other similar entities.
- ❖ Knowledge of energy will help nurses to understand the use of energy in body functioning and the energy requirements of an individual in form of the calories.
- ❖ Nurses understanding the principles of body mechanics can utilize the energy more effectively without putting the body in much strain.

- The knowledge of the levers can help nurses to understand the mechanisms of the simple article used in clinical practices, scissors, forceps; oxygen cylinder carrying stands and so many other clinical articles.
- Knowledge of levers helps nurses understand about functioning of the different body joints and plan for physiotherapy exercises.
- Pulleys are used to lift heavy weights to open windows, and move draperies to raise heavy operating room lamps, and other apparatus in the laboratory.
- The chief use of pulleys in therapy is in balanced traction.
- Pulleys are used in the rehabilitation of patients to prevent atrophy of muscles and joints to restore motion.

QUESTIONS

Q.1: Why does a patient lying in bed for a long time develop sores? State the law that explains it.

Q.2: Explain the principles of simple machine, different types of simple machine and their applications.

Q.3: Give examples of anatomical lever and pulley in the human body.

Q.4: Traction is used in the treatment of some fractures. Explain it.

Q.5: Discuss the principles of force, energy and work in nursing.

BIBLIOGRAPHY

1. Alekseev GN. Energy and Entropy. Moscow: Mir Publishers, 1986.
2. Corbell HC, Stehle P. Classical Mechanics New York: Dover Publications, 1994: 28.
3. Coulomb C. "Recherches théoriques et expérimentales Sur La Force de torsion et Sur L'élasticité Des fils de metal". Histoire de l'Académie Royale des Sciences, 1784.
4. Cutnell J, Johnson KW. Physics, (6th edn). Hoboken, NJ: John Wiley & Sons Inc, 2004.
5. Drake S. Galileo At Work. Chicago: University of Chicago Press, 1978.
6. Duffin. Electricity and Magnetism, (3rd edn). McGraw-Hill, 1980.
7. Feynman RP, Leighton RB, Sands M. Lectures on Physics, Vol 1. Addison-Wesley; Kleppner, Daniel; Robert Kolenkow). An Introduction to Mechanics. McGraw-Hill, 1973.
8. Feynman, Leighton Sands. The Feynman Lectures on Physics. The Definitive Edition Volume II. Pearson Addison Wesley, 2006.
9. Halliday RD, Krane KS. Physics V. 1. New York: John Wiley & Sons, 2001.
10. Henderson T. "The Physics Classroom". The Physics Classroom and Mathsoft Engineering & Education, Inc. 2004.

11. Hetherington NS. Cosmology: Historical, Literary, Philosophical, Religious, and Scientific Perspectives. Garland Reference Library of the Humanities, 1993.
12. Land H. The Order of Nature in Aristotle's Physics: Place and the Elements, 1998.
13. Lofts G, O'Keeffe D, et al. "11-Mechanical Interactions". Jacaranda Physics 1 (2 edn.). Milton, Queensland, Australia: John Willey & Sons Australia Ltd. 2004.
14. Newton I. The Principia Mathematical Principles of Natural Philosophy. Berkeley: University of California Press, 1999.
15. Parker S. Encyclopedia of Physics, Ohio: McGraw-Hill, 1993: 443.
16. Rashed R. "The Celestial Kinematics of Ibn al-Haytham", Arabic Sciences and Philosophy. Cambridge University Press, 2007.
17. Serway RA, Jewett JW. Physics for Scientists and Engineers (6th edn). Brooks/Cole, 2004.
18. Smil V. Energy in nature and society: general energetics of complex systems. Cambridge, USA, 2008.
19. Smith C. The Science of Energy—a Cultural History of Energy Physics in Victorian Britain. The University of Chicago Press, 1998.
20. Tipler P. Physics for Scientists and Engineers: Mechanics (3rd edn). New York: W.H. Freeman, 1991.
21. Tipler P. Physics for Scientists and Engineers: Mechanics, Oscillations and Waves, Thermodynamics (5th edn). WH Freeman, 2004.
22. Verma HC. Concepts of Physics, Vol. 1, Bharti Bhavan, 2004.
23. Walding R, Rapkins G, Rossiter G. New Century Senior Physics. Melbourne, Australia: Oxford University Press, 1999.
24. Wandmacher C, Johnson A. Metric Units in Engineering. ASCE Publications, 1995.
25. Awrejcewicz, J. (2012). Fundamental Principles of Mechanics. In: Classical Mechanics. Advances in Mechanics and Mathematics, Vol 28. Springer, New York, NY. https://doi.org/10.1007/978-1-4614-3791-8_1
26. Karel Velan, A. (1992). Gravitation. In: The Multi-Universe Cosmos. Springer, Boston, MA. https://doi.org/10.1007/978-1-4684-6030-8_10
27. Alrasheed, S. (2019). Newton's Laws. In: Principles of Mechanics. Advances in Science, Technology & Innovation. Springer, Cham. https://doi.org/10.1007/978-3-030-15195-9_3

CHAPTER 5

Heat

Navjot Kaur, Suresh K Sharma

Chapter Outline

- Nature of Heat
- Measurement of Heat
- Transfer of Heat
- Effects of Heat on Matter
- Relative Humidity
- Specific Heat
- Temperature Scales
- Regulation of Body Temperature
- Use of Heat for Sterilization
- Application of Heat Principles in Nursing

■ INTRODUCTION

Healthcare practices are using heat and cold applications for several years for benefiting the patients suffering from several kinds of disorders. One can witness nurses providing hydrotherapies to patients having raised body temperature. Similarly, heat application has been empirically proved to be beneficial for the management of arthritis, sprains, contusions, sinusitis and back pain, etc.

■ NATURE OF HEAT

To understand the nature of heat, let us consider a cup of hot tea. From experience, we know that tea will lose energy (heat) and get cooled. Similarly, you may consider rubbing palms. The work done in rubbing produces warmth (heat). So we can say that heat is associated with the flow of energy. That is, it is energy in transit. In terms of atoms/molecules of a system (or material) we can say that:

"Heat is intimately connected with motion; it is the total kinetic energy of molecules/atoms making up a system".

How do we decide the direction of heat flow from one body to another? Before we answer this question, you should do a simple activity. "Take three cups and put hot water in one (say, cup no.1), water at room temperature in the second (say, cup no. 2), and cold water in the third (say, cup no. 3). Put your left hand in cup no.1 and your right hand in cup no. 3. Now shift both hands to the cup no. 2. How do you feel? Your left-hand feels that cup no. 2 contains cold water (heat flowing from the hand with water) while right-hand feels that the same cup (that is, cup no. 2) has hot water (heat is flowing from the water to the hand). This activity shows that we cannot rely on our senses for deciding the direction of flow of heat energy. We must look for a more precise parameter.

A quantitative measure of heat/thermal energy of the system is given by temperature. It determines the direction in which heat energy is transferred from a system when it is placed in contact with another. (It arose from the physiological sensation of hotness.) For example, when we touch a hot cup, our fingers register a feeling of warmth physically; it means that the energy is flowing from the cup to our fingers. The cup is said to be at a higher temperature than the finger (which is at 98.6°F). We may, therefore, conclude that:

"Temperature characterizes the thermal state of a body and determines whether energy will flow from or towards it from another body in thermal contact".

Heat and temperature are not the same in nature:
- Heat is the total energy content of a system, whereas temperature is a measure of this energy and decides the direction of the flow of energy.
- You can imagine that heat is analogous to the quantity of water. Can you think of a similar astrology of temperature? It is analogous to the level of water.
- Two bodies having the same temperature can have different quantities of heat. For example, a spoonful of a sweet liquid taken from a jug is as sweet as the liquid in the jug, though it does not contain as much sugar. Similarly, the temperature of boiling water in a tea cup may be the same as that in a big bucket, but the heat content of the water in the bucket will be much greater.

■ MEASUREMENT OF HEAT
- As a form of energy, heat has the unit joule (J) in the International System of Units (SI). However, in many applied fields in engineering, the British thermal unit (BTU) and the calorie are often used.

The standard unit for the rate of heat transferred is the watt (W), defined as one joule per second
- ❖ Quantity of heat is defined as the sum of the kinetic energy of all the molecules of which an object is composed of.
- ❖ The temperature of an object is a measurement of the speed of its molecules (i.e. hotness).
- ❖ Any form of energy that increases the speed of the molecules of an object will raise the temperature of the object. For example, if the pitcher of water is heated by a gas flame or by an electric hot plate, energy is transmitted from the gas flame or the hot plate to the molecules of the water in the pitcher. The resulting increase in the temperature of the water is actually due to the increase in the motion of the molecules of water.
- ❖ You can get an idea about the body temperature of a person by your sense of touch. In this case, your hand acts as a temperature sensor and compares the person's body temperature with yours. But this method is not reliable; it provides only a qualitative measure. To get a better measure of temperature, we must know to express it quantitatively. The device that gives a quantitative measure of temperature is called a thermometer. The earliest thermometer was developed by Galileo.
- ❖ In a thermometer **(Fig. 5.1)**, we make use of some temperature-dependent and measurable properties like length, volume, or electrical resistance of matter. We know that most substances expand when heated and contract when cooled. In principle, any such substance could be used as an indicator in a thermometer. But the most commonly used substance in an ordinary thermometer is mercury. However, nowadays uses of mercury thermometer is banned in a healthcare setting due to their deleterious effects on health and therefore digital thermometer is recommended for clinical uses.

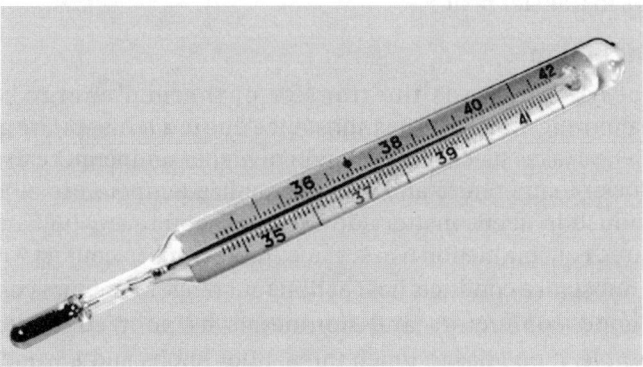

Fig. 5.1: Thermometer.

Advantages of Mercury as the Thermometric Substance

- Mercury is easily visible through glass because it is opaque to light.
- It can conduct heat rapidly.
- It does not wet glass.
- It has a low freezing point and high boiling point so that the range of temperature for which it is used is large.
- It expands uniformly with rise in temperature.

Construction of Mercury Thermometer

A typical thermometer consists of a thin-walled glass bulb, attached to a capillary tube of the uniform bore. The bulb and capillary tube are filled with mercury and heated to a temperature a few degrees above the maximum temperature thermometer is designed to measure. The mercury rises in the tube and overflows. The open end is then sealed. The tube is now marked with reference points called fixed points. These points are usually the position of the mercury in the tube when it is placed in melting ice (lower fixed point) and steam (upper fixed point). The intervening distance between these two fixed points is then graduated into a number of equal intervals, and a scale is thus devised.

■ TRANSFER OF HEAT

Heat can be transferred from one surface to another in several ways. We now know that when an object is at a temperature higher than its surroundings; energy is transferred to the surroundings. This is analogous to the flow of fluid from a region of higher pressure to a region of lower pressure. The human body uses a variety of mechanisms to transfer heat produced due to various internal functions of the body and maintain an average temperature of 98.6°F. In the same way, the skin of the whole body also loses heat by conduction, convection, and evaporation. Following are the main ways to transfer heat.

Conduction

Heat conduction is the transfer of thermal energy between neighboring molecules in a substance due to a temperature gradient. It always takes place from a region of higher temperature to a region of lower temperature and acts to equalize temperature differences. Conduction needs matter and does not require any bulk motion of matter. For conduction two surfaces must come in contact with other.

Substance conducts heat at different rates. Metals are considered as good conductors and nonmetals as poor conductors. For example, if one has to touch metal door knobs and a wooden door simultaneously on a cold day, the metal knob would feel much cooler than the wooden door. This sensation is due to the ability of metals to conduct heat from the body much more rapidly than wood.

Applications of Conductors

- Mercury is a good conductor of heat. So it expands rapidly with a slight increase in temperature.
- Conductors play an important part in nursing and therapeutics. When it is necessary to release heat slowly to an external portion of the body, a poor conductor is used. Rubber is one such poor conductor. It conducts heat more slowly than does a metal. Therefore, it is used in the manufacturing of hot water bottles, icecaps, and ice collars.
- Air, which is a mixture of gases, is a poorer conductor than rubber. A layer of air between a piece of equipment and the body acts as an insulator to prevent heat from passing too rapidly. So a hot water bottle is usually placed in a cloth cover such as flannel, which encloses a layer of air that separates the hot water bottle from the patient. The air slows the passage of heat energy, prevents burning the patient, and prolongs the therapeutic effect.

Convection

This mode of transfer of heat is possible in fluids (liquids and gases) and that too is because of gravity. When a fluid is heated, the hotter part expands, and the density of this portion of the liquid decrease. Due to the buoyancy force; the hotter part, being lighter, tends to rise and its place is taken by the colder and heavier fluid from the top and sides. This, in turn, gets heated and rises up, and so on. *The movement of the hotter part of the liquid upwards and the colder part towards the bottom constitutes the convection current and the transfer of heat due to this process is called convection.*

    This can easily be seen by coloring water by keeping a crystal of potassium permanganate at the bottom of the flask. During pathological testing of urine using a spirit lamp and test tube we can observe the, effect of convection. So we can say that: *In convention, heat is transferred by the actual movements of matter.*

    The process of convection is entirely different from conductions where heat energy is transmitted by atoms/molecules via collisions without being drifted. Some familiar examples of convection are given below:

- You must have seen the rising smoke up a chimney of oil lamps: Hot air above the flame rises up the chimney, its place being taken by cold air from below drawn from the room.

- Wind blows due to convection currents set up in the atmosphere due to, unequal heating of land and sea breezes, and trade winds are caused by convection currents in the atmosphere.
- The effectiveness of ventilation in our homes, hospitals, and public buildings depends upon convection currents.
- For clinical purposes, a thermos bottle is used and a sedative bath is prescribed to help emotionally disturbed patients.
- Steam inhalations and colonic irrigations transfer heat by convection.
- Natural convection and anomalous expansion of water play a very important role in saving the lives of aquatic animals when the atmospheric temperature goes below 0°C on winter days. When water at the surface is cooled, it becomes denser and goes down. Less cold water from the bottom, comes up to the surface and gets cooled and so on. This way the entire water is cooled to 4°C. Further, water at the surface gets cooled; it expands and its density decreases. So, it remains on the surface only and gets cooled further, and then it starts freezing. As ice is a poor conductor, so freezing to downwards is very slow and the temperature at the bottom remains 4°C for long times.

Radiation

Heat is transferred from the sun to the earth without requiring any material medium. Heat energy can be transmitted through a vacuum from some source of heat. The process of emitting energy is called the radiation of an object. Highly polished objects, such as a mirror and light-colored objects reflect radiant energy. For example, the use of lasers.

Evaporation

Heat from the human body is also lost through breathing, by perspiration, by urination, by defecation and through exposed body parts. Loss of heat in these processes is due to evaporation or vaporization. Vaporization takes places in all liquids due to the movement of molecules from the liquid surface. The slow and spontaneous change from the liquid to the vapor or gaseous state of matter is called evaporation. As evaporation takes place, it results in cooling. The use of ecu-de-cologne on your body gives a cooling sensation due to evaporation.

A newborn baby loses (transfers) heat by all four mechanisms **(Fig. 5.2)**.

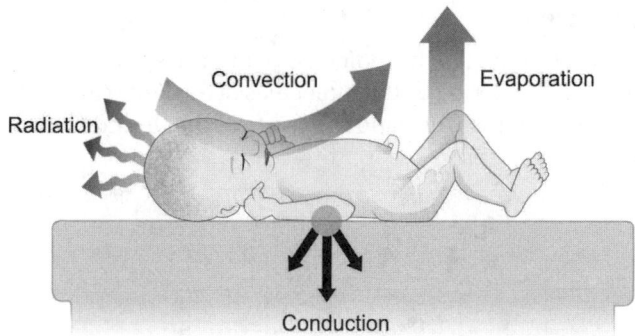

Fig. 5.2: Illustration on different Modes of Heat Transmission.

■ EFFECTS OF HEAT ON MATTER

There is known effect of heat of different matters like with lower temperature liquids change in solid and with increased temperature solid changes to liquid or gases. Following are some of the physical technicalities need to learn to understand the effect of heat on different matter.

Freezing and Melting Points

The temperature at which a liquid changes to a solid is called its freezing point. The temperature at which the same solid is changed back to a liquid is its melting point **(Fig. 5.3)**.

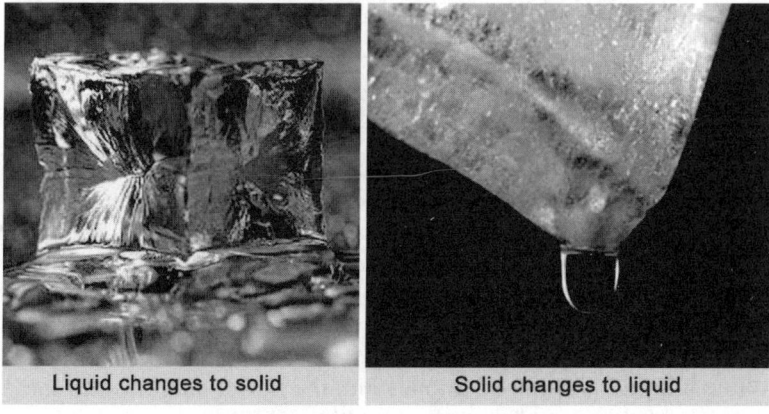

Fig. 5.3: Freezing and melting points.

Vapor Pressure

When a liquid is heated, its molecules leave the surface of the liquid. The pressure developed by the molecules of the liquid as it is changed into a gas is known as the vapor pressure of that liquid **(Fig. 5.4)**.

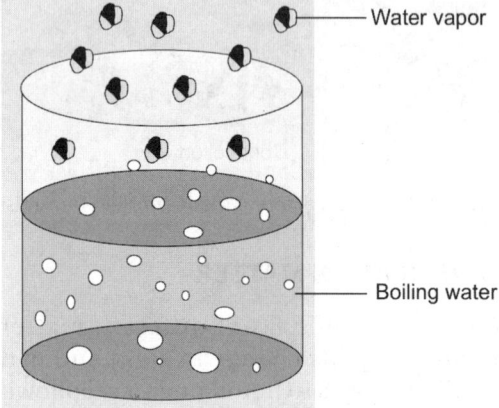

Fig. 5.4: Vapor pressure.

Boiling Point

The boiling point of a liquid is the temperature at which its vapor pressure is equal to atmospheric pressure. A certain quantity of heat is absorbed by the molecules of a liquid when it changes from a liquid to a vapor at the boiling point, this same amount of heat is lubricated when the vapor (gas) condenses to a liquid. The boiling point of water is 100°C.

Heat of Fusion

The heat of fusion is the number of calories needed to produce molecular separation so that material will pass from the solid to the liquid state at the melting point. When ice changes into water at 0°C, approximately 80 calories of heat are absorbed before the ice melts to form 1 gm of liquid water. Ice-filled caps and collars are effective is reducing fever because of the heat of fusion of ice.

Heat of Solidification

When a liquid is changed into a solid, the liquid liberates the same number of calories, that is absorbed in changing from a solid to a liquid. Water releases 80 calories when 1 gm of water is at 0°C changes to ice at the same temperature.

Heat of Vaporization

The number of calories needed to change 1 gm of liquid at a particular temperature to a vapor (gas) at the same temperature is called the heat of vaporization of that substance. The heat of vaporization of water is about 538 cal/gm at 100°C.

Heat of Condensation

When steam at 100°C condenses to form water at 100°C it liberates the heat absorbed when it is changed from a liquid at 100°C to a gas at 100°C. The heat of condensation is the number of calories liberated when a gas condenses to form 1 gm of a liquid at a particular temperature.

Heat of Combustion

It is the quantity of heat in calories given off during the combustion of 1 gm of a substance. It is also measured in kcal/gm.

Sublimation

It is a direct change from the solid to the vapor phase. Dry ice (solid CO_2), camphor, iodine and naphthalene passes directly from the solid to the gaseous phase.

■ HUMIDITY

The concentration of water vapor present in the air is known as humidity. The widely employed primary measurements of humidity are: absolute humidity, relative humidity and specific humidity

Absolute Humidity

Absolute humidity describes the water content present in the air and is expressed in either grams per cubic meter or grams per kilogram. The absolute humidity in the atmosphere ranges from near zero to roughly 30 grams per cubic metre.

Mathematically absolute humidity is defined as mass of the water vapor divided by the volume of the air and water mixture, which is expressed as

The absolute humidity varies with respect to air temperature and pressure changes, if the volume is not fixed. The mass of water vapor per unit volume in the equation is also defined as volumetric humidity.

Relative Humidity

The relative humidity of an air water mixture is defined as the ratio of the partial pressure of water vapor in the mixture to the equilibrium vapor pressure of water over a flat surface of pure water at a given temperature. It is normally expressed as a percentage. Higher percentage indicates that the air-water mixture is more humid.

Relative humidity is a crucial metric that is used in weather forecasts as it is an indicator of the likelihood of precipitation, dew or fog. In hot summer weather, a rise in relative humidity increases the temperature of humans by hindering the evaporation of perspiration from the skin. Relative humidity is expressed as a percentage. For example, if relative humidity on a given day (that is, at a given temperature) is 60%; it means that 60 units of water vapors are present per cubic meter of air which saturates with 100 units of water vapor.

Importance of Relative Humidity
- A high humidity is maintained in operation theaters as it prevents the drying of the exposed tissues. It also reduces the hazard of explosion due to ether fumes.
- Premature infants also require a high humidity environment so that evaporation from the nasal passage can be minimized. If the air at 68° F has a vapor pressure of 8.7 mm Hg and the normal vapor pressure at 68° F is 17.4 mm Hg and the relative humidity is 50%.

$$\frac{8.7 \, mm \, Hg}{17.4 \, mm \, Hg} \times 100 = 50\%$$

If the same air containing 8.7 mm Hg of vapor pressure were reduced in temperature to 49° F, the relative humidity would be nearly 100%. The temperature at which the existing water vapor that produces saturation is called the dew point. A slight decrease in temperature below this point may produce a condensation of water vapor in the form of dew or frost.

Specific Humidity
The ratio of mass of the mass of water vapor to the total mass of the air parcel is known as specific humidity

■ SPECIFIC HEAT
The specific heat of a substance denotes the amount of heat required to raise the temperature of a unit mass of a substance by 1°C.
- Specific heat of a substance is the ratio of its thermal capacity to that of water at 15° C.
- If the thermal capacity(s) of a substance is known, the heat (H) necessary to change temperature of mass (m) from an initial

temperature (t_1) to a final temperature (t_2) can be calculated by the following formula:

H = ms (t_2-t_1) or H = msDt

Since by definition the thermal capacity of water is 1, specific heat is quantitatively equal to the thermal capacity. The thermal capacity of common substances is given in **Table 5.1**.

Table 5.1: Thermal capacity of common substances.

Substance at 20°C	In cal/gm/ °C/ BTU/ lb/ °F
Blood (37°C)	0.80
Water	1.00
Alcohol	0.58
Mercury	0.03
Ice	0.51

■ TEMPERATURE SCALES

Two commonly used scales for measuring temperature are **(Fig. 5.5)**:
- The Fahrenheit scale, which was devised by German scientists Gabriel Heit (1714).
- The Celsius scale (also called the Centigrade scale). The Celsius scale was proposed by a Swedish scientist, Anders Celsius (1742).

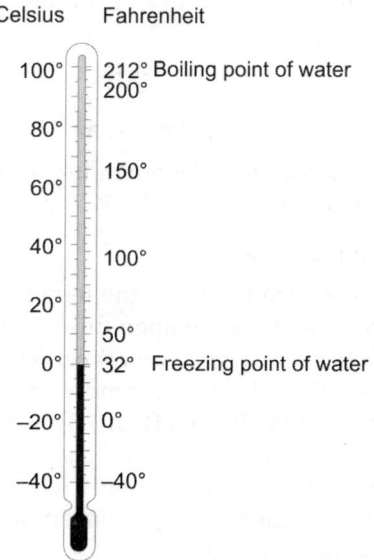

Fig. 5.5: Celsius and Fahrenheit scale.

- On Celsius scale, the freezing point of water is 0° and the boiling point of water is 100°. The interval between the two fixed points is divided into one hundred equal parts.
- In the Fahrenheit scale, the freezing point of water is 32° and the boiling point of water is 212°. The interval between the two fixed points is divided into 180 equal parts.
- Thus, 32°F = 0°C and 212°F = 100°C. Clearly, the Celsius scale is more convenient.

$$\frac{F-32}{C-0°} = \frac{212-32°}{100-0°} = \frac{180°}{100°} = \frac{9}{5}$$

- In order to convert a reading of temperature from one scale to the other, following equation is used:

$$\frac{F-32}{9} = \frac{C}{5}$$

By this equation, the human body temperature of 98.6°F corresponds to 37°C.

- Besides the Fahrenheit and Celsius scales, the absolute or Kelvin scale is also used in physics. The lowest fixed point on this scale is known as absolute zero, which is equivalent to −273°C (−459.6°F) conversions from the absolute scale, i.e. in K, to the Celsius scale is:

$$C° = K - 273$$

Whereas, the conversion from the Celsius scales to the Kelvin scale is:

$$K = C° + 273$$

Relation between Celsius Fahrenheit and Kelvin scales

In order to convert a reading of temperature from one scale to the other, following equation can be used OSC Equation:

Clinical Thermometer

This thermometer is used to record the temperature of the body. In a clinical thermometer, the temperature is recorded in degrees Fahrenheit (or degrees Celsius). In very precise thermometers, each degree is further subdivided into two or more equal parts. Parts of the clinical thermometer are as follows **(Fig. 5.6)**:

- The stem of the thermometer usually has a curved surface that magnifies the numbers on the scale and a flat surface that prevents it from rolling. A white backing is placed behind the mercury column to make reading easier.

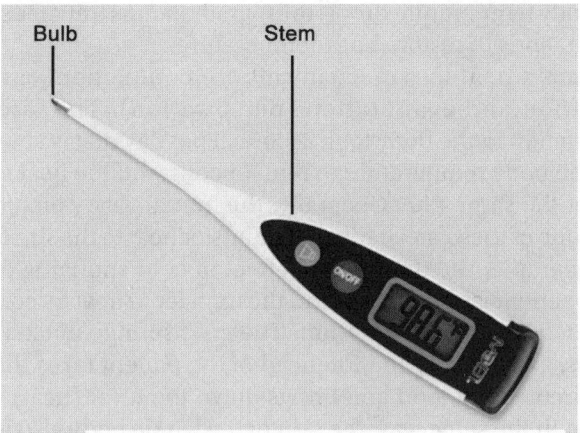

Fig. 5.6: Oral thermometer.

- Oral thermometers are usually made with a long, slender *bulb*, so the mercury in the bulb is exposed to a large surface, the mercury absorbs heat rapidly and registers quickly is a maximum reading thermometer. This means that the column of mercury continues to show the maximum.
- Rectal thermometers have a shorter, thicker-walled bulb and register more slowly than oral thermometers.
- The clinical thermometer temperature level even remains the same after use. So, before using it again, it is reset by shaking the mercury down into the bulb. This is made possible by constriction in the bore of the tube immediately above the bulb.

■ REGULATION OF BODY TEMPERATURE

- Basal metabolism of the body causes heat production. Over and above the basal metabolism, there are other factors that contribute to heat production in the body. A healthy body functions best at an internal temperature of about 37°C (98.6°F). But everyone has their own individual "normal" body temperature, which may be slightly higher or lower. Our bodies also constantly adapt their temperature to environmental conditions. It goes up when we exercise, for instance. And it is lower at night, and higher in the afternoon than in the morning.
- Our internal body temperature is regulated by hypothalamus. The hypothalamus checks our current temperature and compares it with the normal temperature of about 37°C, when body temperature increases, due to heavy exertion: the hypothalamus initiates sweating and vasodilatation. On the other hand, when

the body temperature drops, the hypothalamus initiates shivering, which tends to restore body temperature.
- The main heat loss mechanisms are conduction, convection, radiation and evaporation (perspiration). The rate of heat production in the body for a 2400 kcal per day diet is about 120 W. For the body temperature to remain constant, the heat should be lost at the same rate. Generally, the human body employs more than one of these mechanisms to transfer heat to the surroundings.
- For example, the therapeutic effect of cold sponging for a high fever patient is achieved due to the transfer of heat by conduction, convection, and evaporation. The cold sponge placed over the groins, axilla, neck, and forehead of the patient takes the heat off the circulating blood and brings down the fever (heat) to a safer range. In the same way, the skin of the whole body also loses heat by conduction, convection, and evaporation.
- The temperature of the human body is the result of a balance between heat energy produced and heat energy is lost. Heat energy is produced in the body mainly due to the oxidation of foodstuffs in the tissues, and the heat energy is lost from the body by conduction, convection, radiation, and evaporation. If a person weighing 70 kg is sitting quietly at rest, she expends nearly 100 kcal per hour. However, the same person will expend 1100 kcal per hour to walk up a flight of stairs. The expenditure of energy for various activities is given in **Table 5.2**.

Table 5.2: Relative expenditure of thermal energy per hour.

Activity	Expended energy
Sitting quietly	1.00
Sleeping	0.65
Lying quietly	0.77
Dressing/undressing	1.18
Typing	1.40
Light exercise	1.70
Walking slowly	2.00
Active exercise	2.90
Severe exercise	4.50
Swimming	5.00
Running	5.70
Walking fast	6.50
Walking upstairs	11.00

- Most of the heat of the body is lost through the skin. The rate at which heat is lost depends on the temperature difference between the skin and the environment. Nearly half of the heat produced in the body is lost by a person sitting comfortably in a room at a temperature of 22°C. This means that even at room temperature, heat loss (mostly due to radiation) is significant.
- The death of a person with heat or sunstroke happens because external heat is applied to the body exceeds the amount normally lost. This upsets the total heat balance of the body and the person collapses.

■ USE OF HEAT FOR STERILIZATION

- Sterilizers are based on the Charles's law that states: the temperature of a gas increases as the pressure increases when the volume is kept constant. The increased temperature of the gas resulting from increased pressure destroys the microorganism. Steam at 100°C in contact with boiling water is called moist heat.
- Nonspore-forming bacteria are killed at from 52 to 70°C; the boiling water is sufficient to kill them, whereas spore-forming bacteria require temperatures from 110 to 72°C to kill them. Hence, 120°C for 30 minutes is the ideal temperature for actual sterilization.
- Sterilizers that are used for sterilizing glassware and powders are based on dry heat. Dry heat with a temperature of 160°C is effective to kill bacteria, but its penetration is less than with steam.
- An autoclave is the equipment used for sterilization of surgical tools and other items.. An autoclave is a device that contains steam in a closed chamber of constant volume and the temperature of the steam is increased. Steam is heated to 121–134°C (250–273°F). To achieve sterility, a holding time of at least 15 min at 121°C (250°F) at 100 kPa (15 psi) or 3 min at 134°C (273°F) at 100 kPa (15 psi) is required. Due to such high temperature of the steam, microorganisms present in the tools kept in autoclaves are destroyed.
- Additional sterilizing time is usually required for liquids and instruments packed in layers of cloth, as they may take longer to reach the required temperature. Following sterilization, liquids in a pressurized autoclave must be cooled slowly to avoid boiling over when the pressure is released.

■ APPLICATION OF HEAT PRINCIPLES IN NURSING

Study of heat and principles of heat helps the nurses to understand:
- Understanding the temperature regulation of the body will help the nurses to understand the basis of pathophysiology of some of the

human disease process such as neonatal hypothermia, heatstroke, frost bite, etc.
- ❖ Use of heat and cold applications in healthcare practices to manage several types of disorders such as fever, arthritis, pain, inflammation, injury, etc.
- ❖ Accurate measurements of the body temperature and working of clinical thermometer.
- ❖ Temperature scales and conversion of one type of temperature scale in another like Centigrade to Fahrenheit Scale or vice versa.
- ❖ Transfer of heat from body to surrounding or vice versa, as well as understand about the regulation of body temperature by losing the heat by different means like conduction, convection, radiation and evaporation.
- ❖ Use of heat in sterilization for effective destruction of microorganisms including spores.
  - **Use in environment preparation:** To prepare the soothing environment in wards and home environmental temperature and humidity is a big concern. Now a days this is maintained by air conditioning units and a nurse should know adequate setting for them. If air conditioning is not available proper ventilation should be maintained, during summer cooler or clay pitcher or any water filled open utensil can be kept to maintain humidity.
  - **Use in care of neonate and old person**
    - Both neonate and old age person are prone to suffer from hypothermia that may lead to pneumonia, so extra care should be taken care while carrying them. For neonate at birth there should be provision of radiant warmer, clothes should be pre-warmed and placed in skin to skin contact of mother as soon as possible.
    - Older people often have diminished temperature sensation and impaired mobility and communication, so they have a tendency to remain in a cool environment. These impairments combined with diminished subcutaneous fat may contribute to hypothermia. For old age person there should be a provision of heater in the room and he or she should wear multilayer cloths instead of single thick cloth as air between layers act as insulator and keep them warm.
  - **Use in care during disease condition**
    - *Hypothermia:* Hypothermia is a core body temperature less than 35°C. This is diagnosed by core temperature by rectal and esophageal probes not by oral temperature, electronic thermometers are preferred. Symptoms progress from

shivering and lethargy to confusion, coma and death. Mild hypothermia requires a warm environment and insulating blankets (passive rewarming). Severe hypothermia requires active rewarming of the body surface with forced-air warming systems, radiant sources and rewarming of core by inhalation of steam, heated infusion and lavage, extracorporeal blood rewarming.

During major surgery, if broad area is exposed and also internal organs are exposed then the nurse should aware about the risk of hypothermia and keep the heater and warm infusion ready.

- *Hyperthermia:* Hyperthermia is defined as a temperature greater than 37.5–38.3°C, (99.5–100.9°F) such elevations range from mild to extreme; body temperatures above 40°C (104°F) can be life-threatening. This can be diagnosed by a clinical thermometer. Symptoms progress from heavy sweating, rapid breathing, fast, weak pulse then hot, dry skin to confusion and aggressive behavior having tachycardia and tachypnea. Eventually, organ failure, unconsciousness and death will result.

  When body temperature is significantly elevated, mechanical cooling methods are used to remove heat and to restore the body's ability to regulate its own temperatures. Passive cooling techniques, such as resting in a cool, shady area and removing clothing can be applied immediately by convention and radiation. Active cooling methods, such as sponging the head, neck, and trunk with cool water, remove heat from the body using latent heat of vaporization and thereby speed the body's return to normal temperatures. Drinking water and turning a fan or dehumidifying air conditioning unit on the affected person may improve the effectiveness of the body's evaporative cooling mechanisms.

  When the body temperature reaches about 40°C (104°F), or if the affected person is unconscious or showing signs of confusion, hyperthermia is considered a medical emergency more aggressive cooling measures are used, including intravenous hydration through cool normal saline gastric lavage with iced normal saline, and even hemodialysis to cool the blood.

- *Pain:* Heat increases the blood circulation and dilates blood vessels in a particular area so prevents ischemic pain. It also softens the proteins in ligaments to provide relief for stiffed joints and muscles. Increased temperature causes increased movement of molecules of applied oil or medication which cause deeper penetration for local effect during massage. It is used in specific disease conditions such as Arthritis, Stiffness of joints and muscles.

Opposite to heat cold application causes shrinkage of blood vessels with decrease in blood circulation to a particular area, so it is used to prevent edema and associated pain as at the intra muscular injection site.

- Heat is used during various procedures such as steam inhalation, normal bath, sitz bath, sponging, sterilization, hot water bottle, infrared lamp, massaging, poultice, rubbing of palms.

■ QUESTIONS

Q.1: Use of bath blanket in bed bath.
Q.2: Effects of steam inhalation in patient with common cold.
Q.3: Why autoclaving is a better sterilization method than simple boiling?
Q.4: Explain difference between heat and temperature. What is the difference between clinical thermometer and laboratory thermometer?
Q.5: Explain the mechanism of temperature regulation by human body and discuss its limitations.
Q.6: Methods of local heating.
Q.7: Running hot water over the medicine bottle metal cap.
Q.8: Heat therapy is given to patients in shock.
Q.9: Use of heat for sterilization.
Q.10: Use of heat in abdominal distension.
Q.11: Sources of heat energy in the hospital setting.

■ BIBLIOGRAPHY

1. Baierlein R. Thermal Physics. Cambridge University Press, 2003.
2. Cengel YA. Boles M. Thermodynamics—An Engineering Approach (4th edn). McGraw-Hill, 2002.
3. Clark, JOE. The Essential Dictionary of Science. Barnes and Noble Books, 2004.
4. Clausius R. The Mechanical Theory of Heat—with its Applications to the Steam Engine and to Physical Properties of Bodies. London: John Van Voorst, 1 Paternoster Row, 1865.
5. Perrot P. A to Z of Thermodynamics. Oxford University Press, 1998.
6. Reif. Fundamentals of Statistical and Thermal Physics. Singapore: McGraw-Hll, Inc, 2000.
7. Schroeder DV. An introduction to thermal physics. San Francisco, California: Addison-Wesley, 2000: 18.

8. Smith JM, Van Ness HC, Abbot MM. Introduction to Chemical Engineering Thermodynamics. McGraw-Hill, 2005.
9. InformedHealth.org [Internet]. Cologne, Germany: Institute for Quality and Efficiency in Health Care (IQWiG); 2006-. How is body temperature regulated and what is fever? 2009 Jul 30 [Updated 2016 Nov 17]. Available from: https://www.ncbi.nlm.nih.gov/books/NBK279457/
10. Osilla EV, Marsidi JL, Sharma S. Physiology, Temperature Regulation. [Updated 2021 May 7]. In: StatPearls [Internet]. Treasure Island (FL): StatPearls Publishing; 2022 Jan-. Available from: https://www.ncbi.nlm.nih.gov/books/NBK507838/

CHAPTER 6

Light

Suresh K Sharma, Navjot Kaur

CHAPTER OUTLINE
- Nature of Light
- Law of Reflection and Refraction of Light
- Lenses
- The Physics of Vision
- Defects of Vision and its Corrections
- Biological Effects of the Light
- Uses of Light in Therapy
- X-rays
- Photosensitivity
- Application of Principles of Light in Nursing

■ INTRODUCTION

Almost all life on earth depends on light. Plants convert light energy into chemical energy via photosynthesis: the most basic foundation of almost all food and life cycles. Along with this, light is responsible for the sense of sight. Light and sound are responsible for our communication with the external world. Just as the ear enables us to apprehend sound waves, the eye is the sense organ that enables us to see the objects around us. Light energy from the external environment is transformed into nerve impulse, which is in turn interpreted in the occipital region of the cerebral cortex. Just as the human body is able to detect and interpret sound waves only within a definite range of frequencies, so it is able to detect and interpret as a vision within a certain range of light waves.

■ NATURE OF LIGHT

The nature of light has been a subject of great interest and research since ancient times. We begin with the historic models for light and then will discuss the modern theory.

Corpuscular Theory of Light

Philosophers of the middle ages imagined that luminous bodies emit a stream of particles or corpuscles that produce the sensation of light when they enter the eye. In line with this point of view, Sir Isaac Newton developed the corpuscular theory of light **(Fig. 6.1)**.

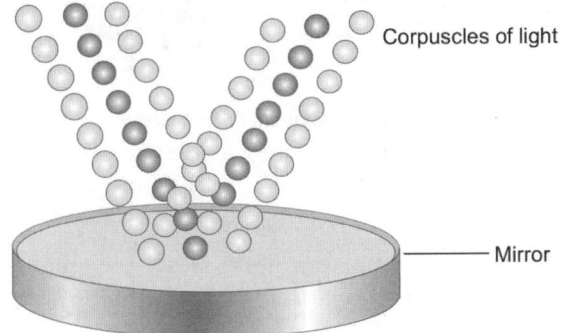

Fig. 6.1: Light as a particle.

Failures of Corpuscle's Theory of Light

These particles travel without being affected by the earth's pull and produce the sensation of light when they enter the eye. But it failed to explain:
* Light bends around corners (diffraction)
* Light travels faster in a vacuum than in a material medium.
* Light redistributes on superposition.

Wave Theory of Light

Huygens conceived the idea that light is transmitted by waves through a material medium. To explain how light waves could pass from the sun to the earth through apparent space: Huygens postulated that hypothetical luminiferous ether filled all of space. He showed that a wave theory of light could also explain reflection and refraction. In 1801, Thomas Young provided a clear demonstration of the wave nature of light, showing that light rays interfere with each other.
* In 1864, Jams Clark Maxwell proposed the electromagnetic theory of light.
* In 1888, Henrich Hertz measured the electromagnetic waves described by Maxwell.
* In 1895, Hendrick Antoon Horentz advanced the idea that the source of electromagnetic light waves are the motion of the electrons in the atoms of elements, and that as the electrons oscillate or revolve, they emit electromagnetic energy of definite wavelength and frequency **(Fig. 6.2)**.

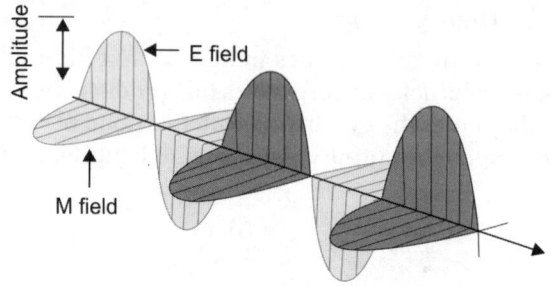

Waves of electromagnetic radiation
Fig. 6.2: Light as a wave.

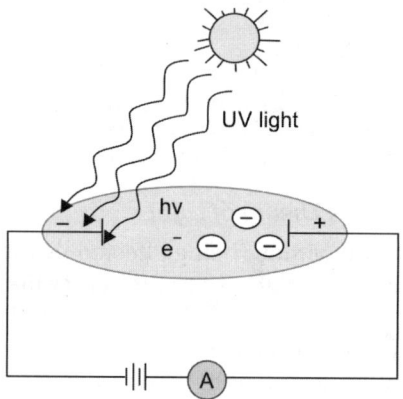

Fig. 6.3: Photoelectric effect.

Failures of Wave Theory of Light

It cannot explain the photoelectric effect. The photoelectric effect is a phenomenon in which ultraviolet light incident on a piece of material causes the ejection of electrons from the surface of the material **(Fig. 6.3)**.

The most remarkable fact about this process is that the energy of electrons emitted by the metal depends on the intensity of the incident light.

Quantum Theory of Light

To explain this, in 1990, Max Planck advanced the quantum theory of light. The quantum theory applied to light waves, states that electron emits energy discontinuously in units of energy called quanta **(Fig. 6.4)**.

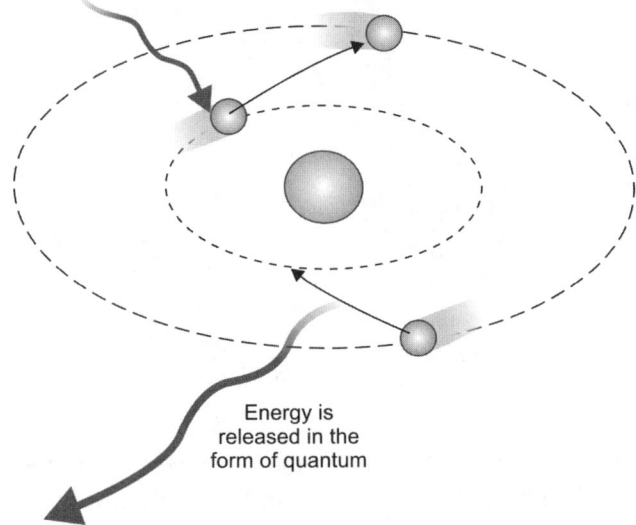

Fig. 6.4: Light in form of quantum.

In 1905, Albert Einstein introduced the use of the term photon, a unit of measurement of quanta of energy. The amount of energy (E) per quantum or photon increases directly as the frequency of light. The frequency (n) may be obtained when the values for velocity of light and the wavelengths are known as

$$n = v/\lambda$$

The energy of a single quantum (photon) is obtained from the following question:

$$E = hn$$

In this relationship, 'h' is known as Planck's constant. It has a value of 6.6256 × 1034 joule- second. For practical purposes, 6.65 × 1034 joule-sec may be used.

If one of these photons is absorbed by an atom of substance, electrons of the atom receive sufficient energy to get ejected from the surface of the substance. The success of Einstein's postulates in explaining experimental observations of the photoelectric effects revealed that light behaves as particles. Thus, you may be tempted to ask how can light behaves as a wave as well as a particle? The answer to this question is yes, light does exhibit dual character. As a wave, it produces interference and diffraction. (These phenomena are not of much interest in medicines) and as particles, it can be absorbed by materials and cause chemical and electrical changes. In fact, the particle character of light is responsible for seeing things when a

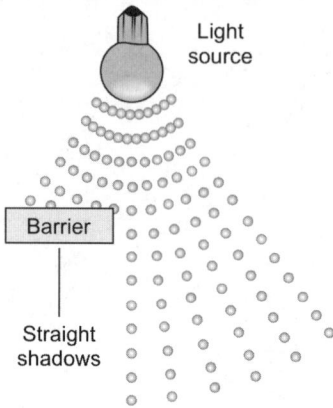

Fig. 6.5: Casting of shadow.

light photon is absorbed in one of the sensitive cells of the retina. Chemical changes in it induce an electrical signal to the brain.

Light at an Interface

Light is invisible, but makes us to see things. Even the act of reading this text involves images made within our eyes. Before we understand the mechanism for seeing things let us learn what is responsible for the formation of images? To explain optical phenomena, like the formation of images; it is sufficient to assume that light travels in straight lines. That is, we can specify the direction of (Light) wave propagation by a straight line. Such a straight line with arrowheads is referred to as a ray of light **(Fig. 6.5)**.

You are familiar with the reflection and refraction of light. These can and should be explained on the basis of the wave nature of light. But for the present, we shall assume that light travels in straight lines and discuss this phenomenon using the concept of rays of light.

By suitable placement of a source of light energy, the object can be made to cast a sharp shadow. This is the most common illustration of the rectilinear propagation of light. A shadow is formed when an opaque object is placed in the path of light. It intercepts the rays of light and the region in space where light does not reach is termed as a shadow.

■ LAW OF REFLECTION AND REFRACTION OF LIGHT

When light falls on the interface separating two media, one or all of the three following processes can occur **(Fig. 6.6)**:
❖ The incident light or a part of it is turned back; that is reflected into the first medium.

CHAPTER 6: Light

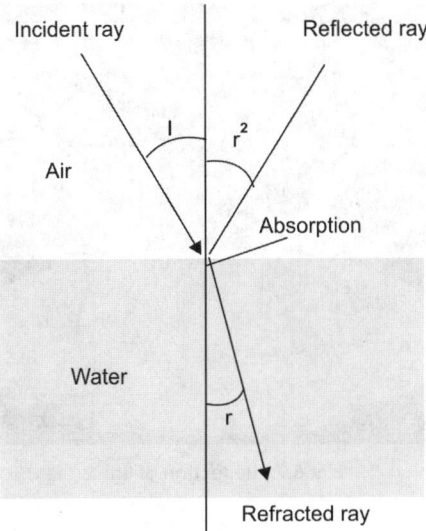

Fig. 6.6: Reflection and refraction of light.

- The incident light is partly or completely absorbed by the second medium.
- A fraction of the incident light is transmitted, i.e. refracted into the second medium as in the case of air-water interface.

Reflection of Light

A light ray is reflected from a smooth surface according to these two laws of the reflection:
- The angle of incidence is equal to the angle of reflection.
- The incident ray, the reflected ray, and normal to the reflecting plane or surface are coplanar.

If you know the angle of incidence, you can predict the direction of the reflected ray using these laws **(Fig. 6.7)**.

The reflection of light from a smooth surface is called specular reflection **(Fig. 6.8B)**. If the surface is rough, the reflecting rays will not be parallel, but in various random directions, such reflection is called diffuse reflection **(Fig. 6.8A)**.

The difference between the two kinds of reflections explains why it is difficult to drive on a rainy night. When the road is wet, the smooth surface of water specularly reflects most of the headlight beams away from our car and when the road is dry, its surface diffusely reflects part of the headlight beams back towards us, enabling us to see the highway clearly.

The process through which light rays fall on the surface and get bounced back is known as a **reflection of light**.

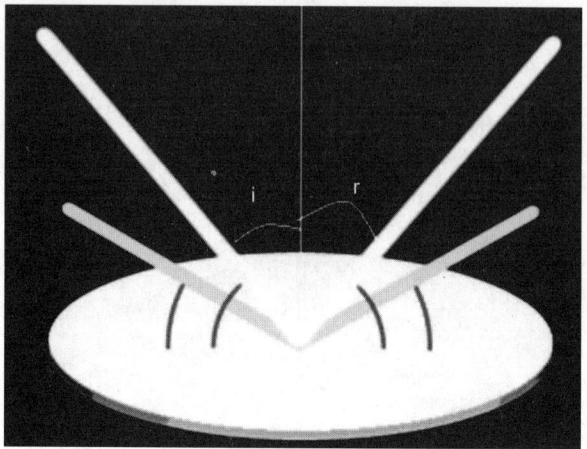

Fig. 6.7: Reflection of light.

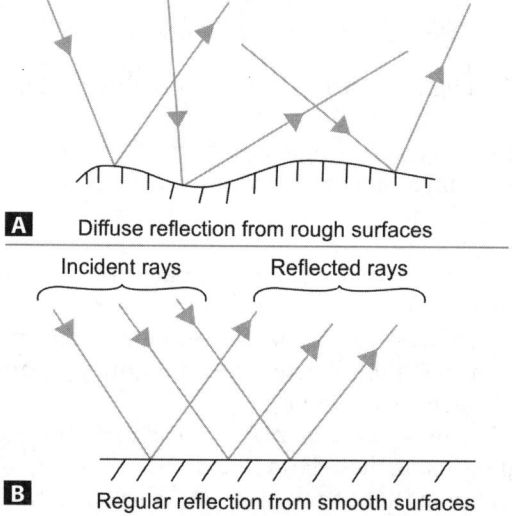

A Diffuse reflection from rough surfaces

B Regular reflection from smooth surfaces

Figs. 12.8A and B: Diffuse and Smooth Reflection of Light.

Types of Reflection

Regular Reflection

The plane mirrors with a smooth surface produce this type of reflection. In this case, the image is clear and is very much visible. The images produced by plane mirrors are always virtual, that is they cannot be collected on a screen.

CHAPTER 6: Light

In the case of curved mirrors with a smooth surface, we can see the images of reflection either virtually or really. That is, the images produced by curved mirrors can be either real (collected on a screen and seen), or virtual (cannot be collected on a screen, but only seen).

Irregular Reflection

Unlike mirrors, most natural surfaces are rough on the scale of the wavelength of light, and as a consequence, parallel incident light rays are reflected in many different directions irregularly, or diffusely. Hence, diffuse reflection helps in seeing the objects and is responsible for the ability to see most illuminated surfaces from any position.

Uses of Reflection

- Reflection is used in periscopes to view advancing enemies on the battlefield from a safe position.
- Reflection is the reason why we see objects.
- Reflection by a concave mirror and a convex mirror has many uses.
- Reflection helps in medical diagnosis and optical communications.
- Light and sound both follow the law of reflection, both being waves.
- Using the law of reflection for sound and light, we can measure the distances accurately to objects.
- Reflection is the reason why we hear the echo of sound.

Refraction of Light

When a ray of light is incident on a plane or surface separating two transparent media, ray bends at the time of changing the medium.

"Refraction is the change in the direction of a wave passing from one medium to another." For a given pair of media (for example air or water) the ratio of the sine the angle of incidence to the sine of the angle of refraction is constant for all angles of incidence. This constant is known as the refractive index of one medium with respect to another. We denote it by the symbol μ.

$$\mu = \sin i / \sin r$$

The above relation is called Snell's law. Since refractive indices of different optical media are different, the speed of light changes when it goes from one medium into another. Thus, an alternative definition of the refractive index of a medium is the ratio of speed of light in a vacuum to its speed in a given medium.

Since velocity of light $c = v\lambda$ refractive indices for lights of different colors will have different values. The value increases from the red end of the visible spectrum to the violet. This suggests that refraction

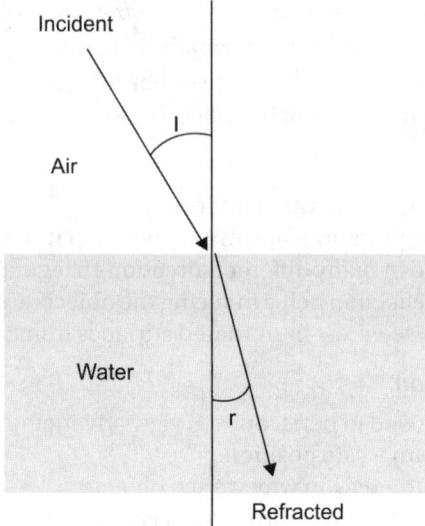

Fig. 6.9: Refraction of light.

index is essentially a property of the medium since velocity of the same light is different in different media.

Refractive index of ordinary glass is 1.3, whereas that of water is 1.5, i.e. glass is denser than the water.

Further, a ray of light bends towards the normal when it goes from a rarer to denser medium **(Fig. 6.9)**. Further extent of bending is a function of wavelength of light. That is why sunlight which consists of seven colors (wavelengths), is split into a spectrum of seven colors when it passes through a prism.

Refraction of Light in Real Life

- Mirage and looming are optical illusions resulting from the refraction of light.
- A swimming pool always looks shallower than it really is because the light coming from the bottom of the pool bends at the surface due to refraction of light.
- Formation of a rainbow is an example of refraction as the sun rays bend through the raindrops resulting in the rainbow.
- When white light passes through a prism it is split into its component colors—red, orange, yellow, green, blue and violet due to refraction of light.

■ LENSES

All of us are familiar with the lenses. We all have lenses in our eyes, some of us have lenses in our spectacles. A lens is made of transparent material and is bounded by two spherical surfaces. Lenses are commonly used to form images via refraction in cameras, microscopes, etc. Light passing through a lens experiences refraction at two surfaces.

Features of Lens

Following are the basic features of the lens **(Fig. 6.10)**:
- **Principal axis/optic axis:** It is a line that passes through the center of curvature of the lens and is perpendicular to the surface.
- **Optical center:** This is a point on the principal axis of equidistance from both surfaces of the lens. Rays of light passing through the optical center do not change their direction and pass through the lens undeviated.
- **Principal focus:** Rays parallel to the principal axis of the lens, after refraction converges to (or appears to diverge from) a point. This point is called the principal focus.
- **Focal length:** The distance from the optical center of the lens to the principal focus.

Lenses and Images

To locate an image made by some object in front of a thin convex lens graphically. Only a few rays need to be drawn through many others exist. The essential rays that are drawn are one along the principal axis, one parallel to it, and one along the secondary axis **(Fig. 6.11)**.

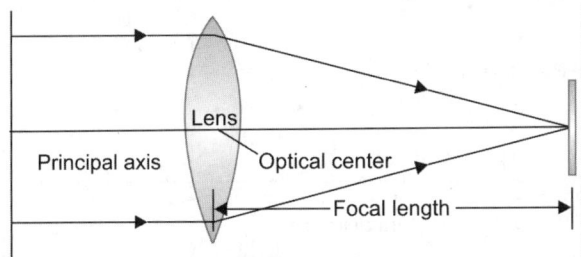

Fig. 6.10: Basic features of a lens

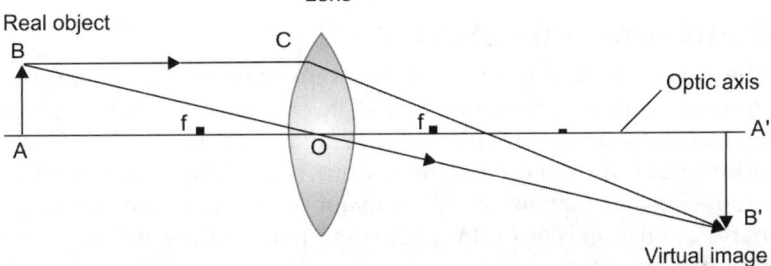

Fig. 6.11: Formation of an image in case of a convex lens.

When an object is placed on the principal axis at a distance from the lens greater than its focal length, (in the diagram object is represented by AB), Ray BC from the tip of the arrow is drawn parallel to the principal axis.

The ray is refracted and passes through the principal focus (FL) to form ray CB'. Another ray (BO) passes through the optical center. It is not refracted and continuous on as ray CB' and OB' meet an image of arrow tip will be formed. If point B' is now connected to the principal axis by a perpendicular line at point A' an image of the arrow will be formed. A screen placed at this point will reproduce on its surface a real and inverted image of the arrow.

In the case of a concave diverging lens, if the source of light is far away and all the rays enter the lens parallel to the principal axis, the rays will be refracted outward and diverge. No real image can be obtained behind the lens was the case with a converging lens, like ray AO is drawn again along the principal axis. Ray BO is parallel to the principal axis. It is bent outwardly and diverges, however from C'D. Ray BO passes through the optical center. In this case, if ray C'D is extended, it meets BO at point B' where the image of the tip appears. As before, if a line is drawn perpendicular from B to the principal axis, the vertical image of the arrow A'B' appears erect and reduced in size **(Fig. 6.12)**.

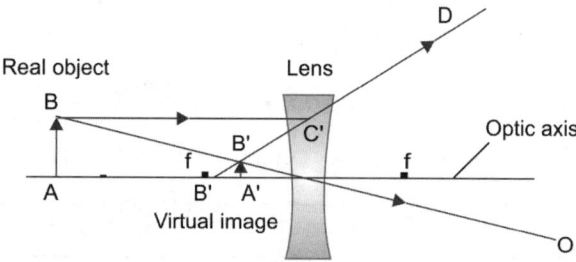

Fig. 6.12: Formation of an image in case of a concave lens.

■ THE PHYSICS OF VISION

The eye is one of the most important human organs. It is responsible for visual contact with nature and all its creations. The helplessness we feel in the dark, particularly in the unfamiliar surroundings, only brings out our dependence on vision. The processes involved in producing the functioning of three major components; the eyes, optic nerves, and visual cortex. In case of dysfunction of any of these parts, blindness results.

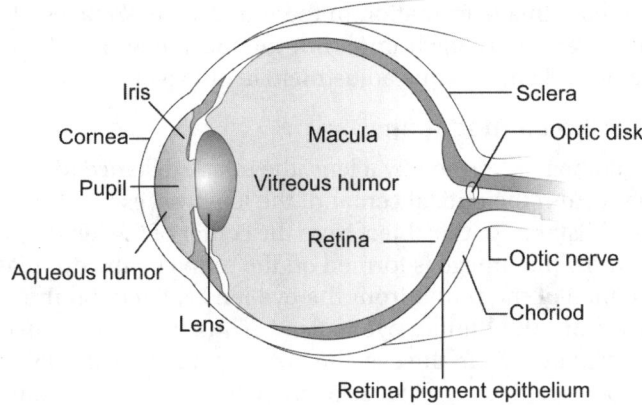

Fig. 6.13: Structure of the eye.

Structure of Eye

The basic components of the structure of the eye are following (**also Fig. 6.13**):

- The eye is like a thick convex lens, which forms images on the retina.
- A white membrane called the sclera covers the eye externally. Its front portion is transparent and more convex than the rest of the eye. It is called the cornea.
- Internal to the cornea is a dark brown membrane called choroids.
- In the front portion of the choroids is a sheath of muscles called the ciliary muscle.
- A circular diaphragm perforated at the center hangs from the ciliary muscles. This diaphragm is called the iris.
- The focusing lens of the eye, which is a biconvex lens is suspended behind the iris. The color of the iris gives color to the eye.
- A purple-red membrane stretches at the internal back portion of the choroids. It is light sensitive and is known as the retina. The retina contains light receptor nerve cells, which receive the light waves.
- The optic nerve fibers carry light sensations from the nerve cells to the visual center of the brain.

The Action of the Eye

Light enters the eye through the hard and transparent cornea into a fluid called aqueous humor. It then passes through the eye lens and vitreous humor via the iris. The combination of the cornea, aqueous humor, lens, and vitreous humor focuses the incoming light on the retina, in the normal eye, the principal focal point coincides with the retina so that all objects are focused on it. The real inverted image formed on the retina is transmitted to the brain. Most of the refraction, which causes image formation in the retina, actually takes place at the cornea and vitreous humor. But the focal length of the lens is adjustable and enables fine adjustment in our vision.

Power of Accommodation

When an image is formed by a lens, the image distance (distance of the image from the optical center of the lens) varies with the object distance (distance of the object from the center of the lens).

We know that image is formed on the retina by the eye lens and the distance of the retina from the eye lens is fixed. So the image distance from the human eye is fixed. Thus to see the objects, at varying distances from the eye, the focal length of the eye lens must change. The change in the focal length of the eye lens is involuntary, the image, however, is always formed on the retina. This capacity of the eye lens to change its focal is called the power of accommodation.

The normal eye can focus on near as well as infinitely remote objects on the retina. The power of accommodation lies in the ciliary muscles, which are connected to the suspensory ligaments in such a way that when the muscles contract, the ligaments relax, releasing the tension on the lens. The lens rounds are in position for near vision and vice versa.

Least Distance of Distant Vision

For every eye, there is a limit to its power of accommodation. This power ceases for objects beyond a certain minimum distance from the eye. The nearest distance up to, which a small object can be seen distinctly, is called the near point of the eye. The distance of the near point from the eye is called the least distance of distant vision. For a normal eye, it is about 25 cm.

We may, therefore, conclude that the human optical system has the following features, which are not available in the most expensive cameras.

- ❖ The eye can observe events over a very large angle even while looking intently at an object directly ahead of it.
- ❖ Blinking provides the cornea with a built-in lens a cleaner and lubricator vision.
- ❖ A rapid automatic focusing system permits viewing objects at far away distances as well as near objects at a short interval.
- ❖ The eye can operate over a wide range of light intensities; daylight and dark light.
- ❖ The eye has a self-regulating pressure system that maintains internal pressure (20 mm Hg) and keeps the eye in shape.
- ❖ The images are blended perfectly giving a good depth perception.

■ DEFECTS OF VISION AND ITS CORRECTIONS

Defects of the vision are as follows:
* Hypermetropia or long-sightedness
* Myopia or short-sightedness
* Presbyopia or far-sightedness
* Astigmatism

Hypermetropia or Long-sightedness or Hyperopia

Hyperopia is a very common refractive condition in childhood and adults. A long-sighted person cannot see near objects distinctly. For long-sighted persons, the distance of near point is greater than 25 cm. This is because the image of an object is placed at the near point from the eye is formed behind the retina.

Conventionally the hyperopia is etiologically classified into:

Axial hyperopia (most common-simple hyperopia): It is due to anterior-posterior axial shortening of the eyeball. Genetic predisposition plays an important role. Retinal edema can cause a hyperopic shift. A 1 mm decrease in axial length leads to 3 diopters of hyperopia.

Curvature hyperopia: It is due to flattening of the cornea or the lens or both. A radius of curvature increases by 1 mm leads to 6 diopters of hyperopia.

Index hyperopia: It is due to the change in the refractive index of the crystalline lens, which occurs in old age or diabetics. The refractory index gradually increases from the center to the periphery.

Positional hyperopia or **absence of the lens (aphakia)** or **ocular pathologic conditions**: This condition occurs due to malposition or absence of the crystalline lens (congenital or acquired) or intraocular lens owing to the creation of an aphakic zone in refractive media. Post-traumatic or post-surgical aphakia is not an uncommon cause of hyperopia.

This defect arises because:
* The eyeball is too short.
* The focal length of the lens is elongated.
* This is normally seen in elderly persons.
* To correct this defect, we interpose a convex lens (converging lens). As a result, the focal length of the combination (eye and lens) decreases and the image is formed on the retina **(Fig. 6.14)**.

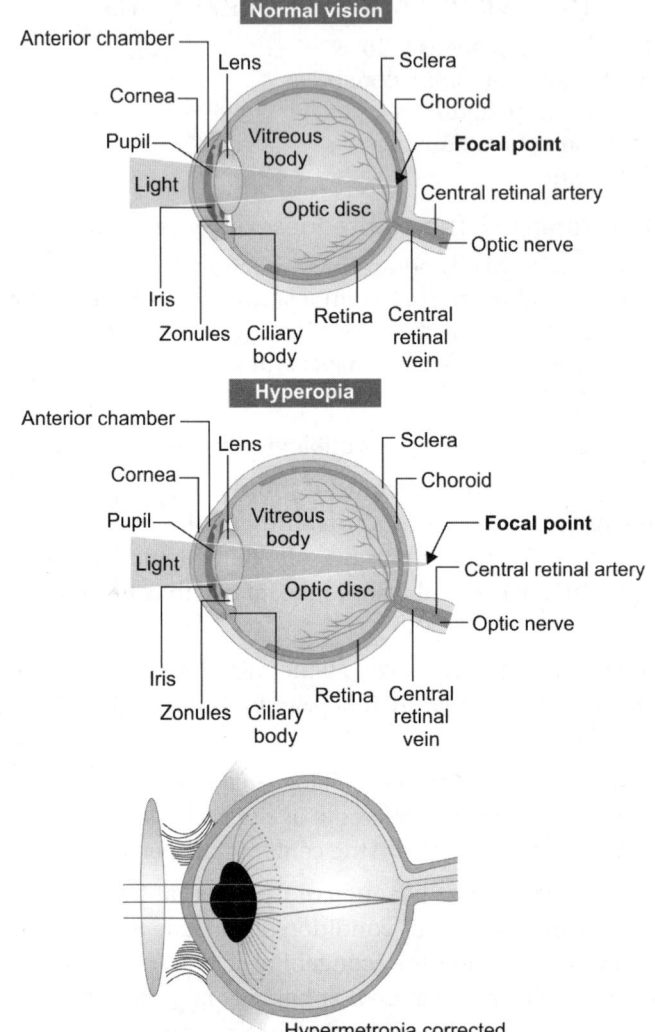

Fig. 6.14: Hypermetropia corrected with a convex lens.

Myopia or Short Sightedness

A shortsighted person cannot see distant objects distinctly. The image is formed in front of the retina.

This defect can arise due to:
- Elongation of the eyeball.
- The focal length of the eye lens is too short.
- It is seen in school or college- going children.
- To correct this defect, a concave (diverging) lens is used **(Fig. 6.15)**.

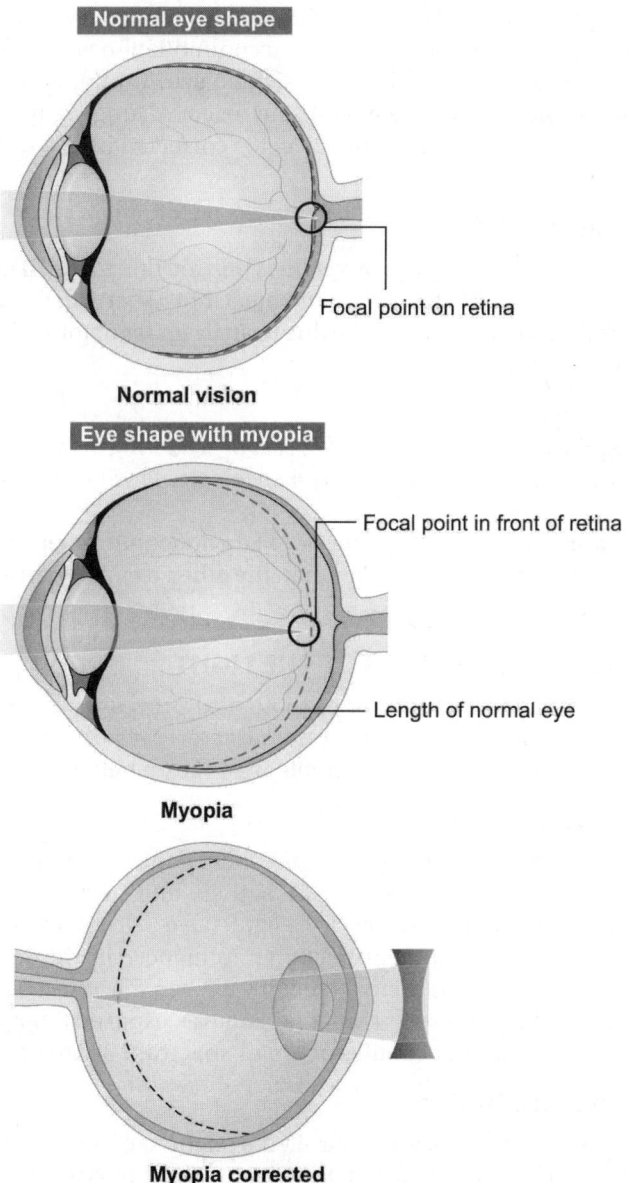

Fig. 6.15: Myopia corrected with a concave lens.

Presbyopia or far Sightedness

This defect is long-sightedness caused due to old age. A progressive decrease in the accommodative capacity of the lens is the major cause of presbyopia. The lenses of the eye, which are crystalline, lose elasticity gradually with age, and the accommodation power of ciliary muscles decreases. Thus, the short-sighted eye in childhood tends to become normal in later years, but the defect of long-sightedness is sure to increase gradually. This defect is corrected by the use of the bifocal lens.

Astigmatism

It is an optical defect, whereby vision is blurred due to the inability of the optics of the eye to focus a point object into a sharp focused image on the retina. This image may be due to an irregular or toric curvature of the lens or cornea.

It is of two types:
1. **Irregular:** It is caused by corneal scar or scattering in the crystalline lens. It cannot be corrected by a spectacles lens but by a contact lens.
2. **Regular:** It is due to a toric surface like a doughnut, where there are two regular radii, one smaller than the other. It can be corrected by a spectacles lens.

■ BIOLOGICAL EFFECTS OF THE LIGHT

Light may regulate a number of biological processes and also the structural as well as behavioural characteristics of animals. The important effects of light on animals are as given below: :

Effect on Metabolism

The absorbed radiant energy heats the tissues and causes protoplasm ionization. This improves enzyme activity and overall metabolic rate. Cave animals, which have little light, have a slower metabolism. The amount of absorption of calcium is influenced by the amount of light to which a person is subjected. It was seen that 15% absorption of calcium was increased when a person was exposed 8 hours daily for 4 weeks to 500-foot candles of broad-spectrum fluorescent light.

Effect on Locomotion

Many lower organisms are controlled by light to control their speed of locomotion (Photokinesis). Studies on blind mussel crab larvae (Pinnotheres maculatus), have shown an increase in swimming speed with increasing illumination. The role of light is often important in orientating locomotion. Phototaxis is the movement of animals in response to light. Positive phototactic is when an animal moves toward the source of light, e.g. Euglena. If it moves away, it is called negative phototactic. (e.g., earthworms, slugs). This can also be noticed that children are active in daytime or in bright light and less active in darkness.

Effect on Development
Some animals have accelerated or retarded development due to light as Salmon larvae develop normally when there is enough light. The absence of light causes abnormal egg development and results in a high mortality rate for larvae. The larvae of Mytilus grow larger in darkness than in the light. The intensity of the light in the environment affects the development of the eyes in many cave-dwelling animals, such as Proteus eyes are either missing or very basic. The eyes of deep-sea fishes and nocturnal animals are larger in size.

Pigmentation Effects
Different light conditions can affect the pigmentation of plants and animals. Due to lack of light, cave animals are often devoid of pigments. Many animals have pigmentation that gives them protection against enemies. This is known as "protective coloration". The body color of a leaf insect is, for example, similar to a leaf. Melanocytes in human skin produce melanin stimulated by Ultraviolet radiations. This is a protective mechanism against further injury to DNA of cells.

Photoperiodicity and Photosensitivity
Photoperiodism is the organism's response to day length. Many organisms have a 24-hour cycle of activity. This is known as diurnal periodicity or circadian rhythm. Photosynthesis, which is subject to fluctuations due to light changes daily, is the most important diurnal rhythm. Copepods, and other planktonic creatures, move toward the surface of the water at night while moving downwards during the day. Some animals are more active in daylight than in darkness, and vice versa. Many organisms' activities in relation to their reproductive cycle are closely related to the moon. This phenomenon is called lunar periodicity. This is when the biological rhythm occurs once or twice per lunar month. Semilunar rhythms occur in 15 days. Lunar rhythms occur in 30 days.

- ❖ Sometimes interaction of light with some chemicals results in toxic substances in the body that may produce a rash. This photosensitizing property is beneficial in the treatment of some skin disorders such as skin cancer, herpes, psoriasis, etc.
  - In the case of malignancy, photosensitizing agents seem to inactivate DNA in unwanted cells.
  - In herpes and psoriasis, these agents inactivate DNA in the protoplasm of causative organisms.
- ❖ Light is effective in treating jaundice in infants.

Influence on Reproduction and Gonads

Light is the key too many animals, including birds, launching their annual breeding activities. In summer, birds' gonads are more active due to increased light. Animals can be classified into short, long, or indifferent day animals. Short-day animals such as deer, sheep, and goats are sexually active during decreased exposure to daylight. Birds that breed in spring experience a lengthening day and are also known as long-day animals. Guinea pigs and squirrels are not affected by daylight. They are therefore indifferent day animals. Light may have a significant influence on the sexual maturity of humans as it has been proven that girls who are blind have an earlier menarche than girls who are normally sighted.

Endocrines: Effect

Evidence suggests that there is a circadian rhythm in the secretion of thyrotrophin-releasing factor and rhythmic variation in ACTH secretion and corticotrophin-releasing factor from the hypothalamus. When rats are continuously exposed to light for a prolonged period of time, the cyclic pattern in gonadotrophins release is eliminated and the normal cycle of the oestrus is replaced with a state of constant oestrus. The constant light stimulus may inhibit the activity of pineal glands, according to some theories. Ultraviolet radiations act on the skin and are effective in the synthesis of vitamin D. In animal experimentation, it is found to inhibit ovulation and modify the secretions of other hormones such as serotonin.

Diapause

A type of dormancy in animals is called diapause. It can occur at any stage of the animal's life cycle, such as egg, larvae, pupa, or adult. Diapause has the same causative mechanisms as plants, i.e. Hormones that are regulated by environmental stimuli.

Below a certain threshold, diapause can occur. Insect to insect, the critical amount of daylight is different. It takes approximately 12 hours for cabbage white butterflies. The pupae go into diapause when the light drops below this level. They do not resume their development until the next spring. Experimentally, it has been proven that light does not stimulate the eyes. Covering them does not stop the diapause response. The light stimulates the brain directly, and possibly produces other substances that inhibit growth-stimulating hormones. In some species, the end of diapause and the transition to longer days could be the most effective stimulant. However, in insects, a certain period of cold is required before growth can be resumed. This is similar to stratification in seeds or buds.

Circadian Rhythm and Health Aspects

Circadian rhythm coordinates a wide variety of body processes, including sleep. The circadian pacemaker is a tiny part of the brain that is strongly influenced by light exposure. Human biology evolved to sleep according to the daily cycles of daylight and darkness. A person's circadian rhythm is closely controlled by sunrise. This allows them to stay awake during daylight hours and sleep when it gets dark. Modern society has many light sources, which can affect the brain's circadian rhythm maker.

The amount of light that we are exposed to each day, as well as the time and duration, can have a significant impact on our sleep quality. Understanding the intricate links between light exposure and sleep will help us to set up our bedroom for consistent, high-quality sleep for patients.

A person's circadian rhythm can be disrupted by excessive or inappropriate artificial light exposure. This can disrupt their sleep and cause other health effects such as eye strain, weight gain, metabolic problems, cardiovascular problems, and even a higher cancer risk. The mood and mental health of people are affected by their circadian rhythms. Seasonal effective disorders, for example, is a form of depression that affects those who live in areas with very short winter months. The winter season can bring about mood changes by reducing daylight.

Melatonin, a hormone naturally produced by the body and closely linked to light. The pineal gland in the brain produces melatonin when it is dark. Light exposure can slow down or stop this production. The hormone is known to increase sleepiness when melatonin levels rise. Daily cycles of melatonin release help to maintain a steady sleep-wake rhythm by normalizing the circadian rhythm. Some people may need synthetic melatonin to regulate their sleep time.

Each sleep cycle has its own characteristics. A person will go through between 70 and 120 minutes of sleep each night. These cycles include multiple stages of sleep, they also include rapid eye movement (REM), and non-REM sleep. Night-time light exposure can slow down transitions between sleep cycles and reduce the quality. Repeated awakenings can disrupt the sleep cycle, resulting in a decrease in time spent in deep, more restorative stages.

Jet lag occurs after long-distance flight travel. Because the body's internal clock remains attuned to the departure time zone, it is most common after crossing five to more time zones. A person might have difficulty falling asleep, wake up early, or feel tired during the day.

Jet lag is usually addressed by adjusting to the new time zone. This can be done by getting sunlight at certain times or avoiding light at other times. This will help to align your circadian rhythm. This can take up to two weeks and may take several days.

Shift workers are often devoid of sleep during the night, which puts them at risk for a misaligned circadian rhythm or the development of shift work disorder. This disorder of the circadian rhythm can lead to insufficient sleep, excessive sleepiness at inappropriate times, mood problems, and increased risk for workplace accidents.

Blue light has a shorter wavelength and is emitted from many LEDs. It has been shown to have a greater effect on melatonin and the circadian rhythm than light that emits a longer wavelength. Many electronic devices such as cell phones, tablets, and laptops emit blue light. This can lead to sleep problems.

Although blue light can be reduced by many phones and tablets, it may still cause sleep disturbances due to stimulation from the screen. Some people are not able or willing to sleep in the darkness. They can use a dim red light source as red light can increase levels of melanin and helps our bodies prepare for bed.

To promote sleep, the first thing that should be done in the bedroom is to make it dark. To create a dark environment, blackout curtains block most of the light from outside. Keep lights dimmed when getting ready to go to bed. A small, low-power lamp may help in the transition to sleep and pitch darkness. Warm color temperature and low illuminance can help to relax and get into the right frame of mind for sleep. Healthy sleep can be supported by routines and habits.

Light therapy is one treatment for many circadian disorders. This involves sitting near a powerful lamp at set times to reset the body's internal clock. To normalize circadian timing, the strong lamp mimics daylight. It is commonly used in the morning. Although all lighting can impact sleep, not all lights have the same effect. Direct sunlight can produce up to 10,000 lux. This is more than bright office lighting, which only rarely exceeds 500 lux. Daylight has a significant influence on sleep and circadian timing. Current studies are being conducted in which human beings are exposed to constant artificial light (absence of normal cyclic exposure) for months. In these cases, the body rhythms become circadian or approximately 24 hours in length.

■ USES OF LIGHT IN THERAPY

The light has significance in medical science.. Some of the common diagnostic and therapeutic uses of light are discussed below (**Fig. 6.16**).

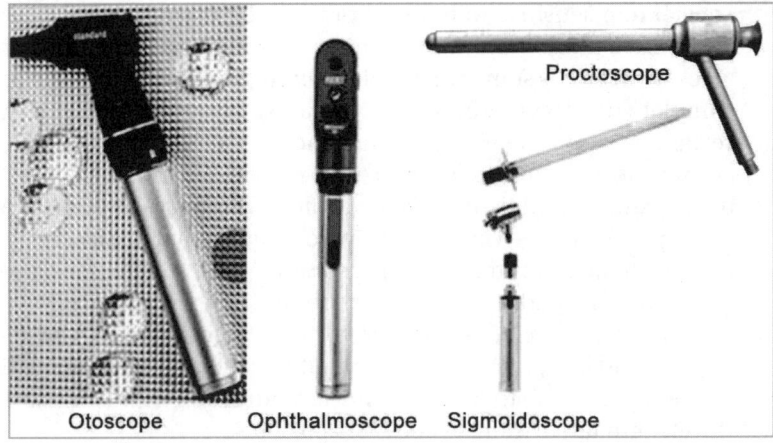

Fig. 6.16: Application of visible light in diagnostic tools.

Visible Light in Medicine

- Visible light is responsible for visual information about the patient, e.g., colors of the skin, to detect the presence of abnormal structures.
- ENT specialist examines internal parts of the ear, nose, or throat by using a curved mirror with a hole in the middle and another lighted instrument called an examination otoscope.
- An ophthalmoscope is used by ophthalmologists for examining the eye.
- Endoscopes-like cystoscopes, proctoscopes, bronchoscopes that are rigid are used to view internal body cavities. Flexible endoscopes by the use of fiber optic techniques are also being discovered. These are mainly used to view the small and large intestines.
- Transillumination (in which light is passed into the body through the skin) is used to study hydrocephalus and pneumothorax in infants. The sinuses, breasts and testes are also examined by this method.
- Visible light is a form of energy and is selectively absorbed by certain molecules. This enables us to use visible light for therapy, particularly in infants, it is successfully used to treat jaundice and maintain their body temperature.

Infrared Radiation

- The transfer of heat energy by radiation from the surface of hot objects is in the form of infrared rays.
- Infrared rays are invisible; penetrate mist, fog, and the tissues of the body better than visible light does.

- Special film sensitive to infrared rays can be used on foggy days to produce photographs. By using visible light, infrared light or black light, as it is sometimes called, photographs can be taken in complete darkness. Infrared photography is especially useful in certain cardiovascular conditions. The light penetrates the skin, permitting the veins under the skin to be photographed.
- Baking lamps used to produce invisible infrared rays in the home or hospital may give visible light and orange light in addition.
- Infrared light is emitted by incandescent lamps, steam pipes, hot stoves, heating pads, and hot water bottles.
- Infrared radiation is classified into two categories mainly near-infrared and far-infrared. Near-infrared radiation has a wavelength range from 700 A to 5,000 A and far-infrared radiation has a wavelength range from 25,000 A to 200,000 A.
- The warmth due to the radiation from the sun is most beneficial for the human body. They can penetrate through the tissues of the body from 1 to 10 mm.
- Infrared radiation heat lamps and heating pads to heat tissues for relieving pain due to muscle ligaments, backache, spondylosis, etc.
- Another clinical application of infrared radiation in medicine is thermography.

Thermography

- It is a method of recording photographically, the heat emitted through the skin at various points on the body (**Fig. 6.17**).
- Thermograph is an infrared camera that in addition to being extremely sensitive to heat emitted by an area of the body is able to transfer heat into an electric current. The current then

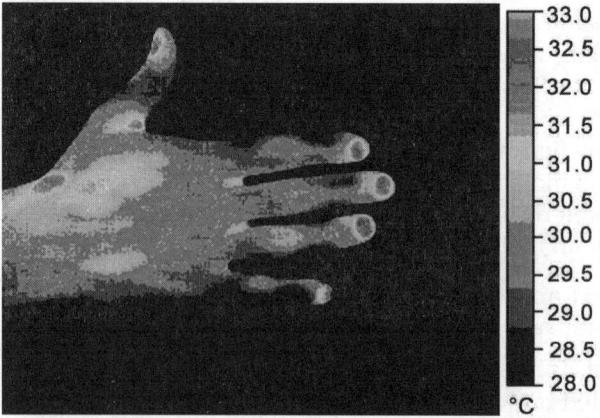

Fig. 6.17: Thermography.

operates a visible light of variable intensity that is recorded on a photographic film. The resulting pictorial representations are called thermographs.
- ❖ Because most tumors have temperatures 1 or 2°C higher than those of surrounding areas, they can be detected by thermography. On the thermogram, the relatively warmer tumor appears lighter in color than the cooler surrounding area.
- ❖ Several principles of physics explain medical thermography. The law that describes the relationship between temperature and radiation is the 'Stefan-Boltzman law'.
  - Total radiations emitted from a surface is proportional to the fourth power of its absolute temperature.
  - Although, variations within the range of 23 to 36°C occur normally.

Uses

- ❖ Diagnosis of tumor and arthritis.
- ❖ Effects of drugs or other agents on the body.
- ❖ In the diagnosis and treatment of rheumatic diseases.
- ❖ Detection of breast cancer and ocular diseases.

ULTRAVIOLET RADIATION

They are basically of two types:
- ❖ Near UV radiation: 2,900 to 3,900 A wavelength.
- ❖ Far UV radiation: 1,800 to 2,900 A wavelength.
  - Both types of radiation are superficial. Both produce chemical changes in the tissues. UV radiations are produced artificially by solids heated to a very high temperature of approximately 3,000°C by either establishing an electric arc between metal and carbon electrodes or by producing glowing mercury vapors.

Uses

- ❖ Production of erythema
- ❖ Exfoliation
- ❖ Activation of ergosterol in the skin to form vitamin D.
- ❖ Bactericidal effects due to changes in the protein molecules of organisms at 2,650 A wavelength.
- ❖ Radiations are also used for sterilization of air using 2,500 A wavelength radiations.
- ❖ It improves general body resistance.
- ❖ In the treatment of rickets and tuberculosis.
- ❖ As a counterirritant in neuritis, lumbago, and fibrositis.
- ❖ In the treatment of skin conditions such as psoriasis, acne vulgaris, etc.

Dangers and Precautions

- Many lamps known as sun lamps produce UV radiation. Their use is prohibited by the Council on Physical Medicine of the American Medical Association because it can cause conjunctivitis and other abnormal conditions of the eye.
- It results from the snow that in bright sunshine reflects a large amount of UVsradiation, electric welding arcs, and other sources of UV rays.
- When UV rays are administered, the eyes of the operator should be protected by clear or dark glasses and the eyes of the patient by pledgets of cotton or gauze moistened with water, which absorbs the radiations.
- Water has an absorption spectrum of 1,800 to 3,000 A in the UV region. This limits the amount of radiation that reaches the organism immersed in water. Similarly, the amount of water vapor in the air limits these radiations from reaching the earth's surface.

■ X-RAYS

- X-rays are electromagnetic waves of an extremely short wavelength of approximately 0.01 nm up to 10 nm and of high frequency.
- They were discovered by roentgen in 1895. He discovered it while he was considering the question of luminescence from the cathode tube with which he was experimenting. He discovered in his studies that an invisible penetrating radiations came from the tube and affected a photographic plate. Because the tube was covered by an opaque shield and because the electron in the tube could not penetrate the glass, he concluded that the unknown radiations were coming from the walls of the tube where the electrons were striking the glass. In addition, because the waves could pass through the glass, roentgen considered these unknown X-rays to be very penetrating. Roentgen further studies on the nature of X-rays led to their use medically within three months after discovery.
- The type of tube used to produce X-rays was refined by Coolidge in 1913. X-rays may be produced in a vacuum tube by the bombardment of a metal target with a stream of electrons moving at high speed. The metal target is usually made up of tungsten or molybdenum. When the electrons strike the target, they are stopped and about 99% of the energy of the electrons is converted to heat. The remaining 1% of energy is converted to X-rays.
- X-rays have great power of penetration and when passed through the body, affect a photographic plate and produce a "negative picture" or a "shadowgraph". Structures and tissues that allow the

rays to pass through them easily appear dark on the developed film and those that do not allow the rays to pass appear as lighter areas on the film.
- X-rays, as it is frequently referred to result from photons of electromagnetic energy. As we know,

$$E = hn$$
$$E = c/\lambda$$
$$\lambda = hc/E$$

So wavelength can be known.

Types

- Hard or high energy X-rays
- Soft or low energy X-rays

The relationship between the energy and wavelength is

$$\lambda = 1/E$$

- So those with high energy are of shorter wavelength and vice versa. Hard X-rays that are used for deep therapy have an average wavelength of 0.14 A. They are generated at about 200 kV. Softer X-rays used for diagnosis or superficial therapy have wavelengths of about 0.7 to 0.5 A and are generated by the voltage of 75 to 100 kV, respectively. The voltage applied in generating the radiations controls the hardness and softness of the X-rays.

Units

The unit of dosage used in X-ray therapy is the roentgen. It is defined as the amount of radiation that the associated corpuscular emission in 1 ml of air at a temperature of 0°C and a pressure of 760 mm of Hg produces in air ions carrying electrostatic units of electricity of either sign. The roentgen refers to ionization produced in the air.

Uses

- When the X-rays pass through the body tissues, ionization of the matter occurs and the position of the electrons within the body tissues changes, producing chemical changes that are destructive to the cells. Cells of malignant tumors are more susceptible to the effect than are the normal cells X-rays are useful in the treatment of superficial lesions of skin cancer and also in irradiatinggdeep-lying tumors of visceral organs.
- When it is necessary tos X-ray the ventricle of the brain, the ventricles are tapped and cerebrospinal fluid is removed. The ventricles are then filled with air. When X-rays are passed through the skull and brain, the air in the ventricles retards their passage and the ventricles are outlined on the photographic plate.

- Certain chemicals such as barium sulfate and diodrast are opaque to X-rays. They are used when it is necessary to outline an organ such as the stomach, kidney or urinary bladder. Since the X-rays do not pass through the organs caused by these chemicals, the organs appear as light shadows on the developed plate.
- By the same principle, air O_2, CO_2, etc. may be injected into the fascial spaces around the kidneys to mark the adrenal glands.
- A miniature radiographic tube for intracavitary insertion has been reported to be used in dentistry to obtain an 'inside-out' wide-angle picture of teeth and jaw.

■ PHOTOSENSITIVITY

It has been seen that administration of dye substances such as methylene blue and other drugs such as quinine to the patients has sometimes resulted in sensitivity reactions to light and possess a potential danger to human life. It is due to the production of the toxic material as a result of the interaction of drugs or dye with light. This phenomenon is known as photosensitivity reactions. An explanation for this reaction is related to the activation of molecules by light energy when a photon of light is absorbed by a molecule, such as dye, energy is transferred to the molecule and raises it to the level of energy above that which it had originally. This increase in energy may appear as heat because of the many collisions of the "activated" molecules with others or the energy may be emitted again from the molecules as another form of light. In still other situations, the molecule may retain the excess energy and remain in the activated state for some time. Most of these reactions are limited to the light of shorter wavelengths. Now in the case of dye, activated dye molecules react with the molecules of the substrate in which they are located (this may be the protoplasm of the cell) to form a substance that is capable of being oxidized. According to one theory, this oxidation product is abnormal and harmful to the organisms and is responsible for the production of symptoms of hypersensitivity **(Fig. 6.18)**.

■ APPLICATION OF PRINCIPLES OF LIGHT IN NURSING

Study of principles of lights nurses will be able to understand:
- Nature of light, will enable nurses to understand the use of light in different healthcare practices.
- Refractive errors of the eye and will understand the corrective measures by using a different type of lenses.
- Use of light in different diagnostic tools like an otoscope, ophthalmoscope, proctoscope, cystoscope and colonoscope, etc.

CHAPTER 6: Light

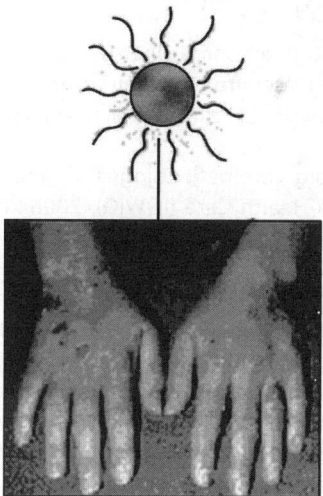

Fig. 6.18: Photosensitivity.

- Use of light in the management of different medical disorders like treatment of malignancies, skin problems, etc.
- Nurses will be able to understand the biological effect of the light on the human body.
- Understand the mechanism of the photosensitivity.

■ QUESTIONS

Q.1: Write two applications of infrared rays in nursing practice.

Q.2: Define power of accommodation. Name the defect of vision related to it and how it is corrected.

Q.3: Use of laser in the repair and treatment of detached retina.

Q.4: Diverging lens to treat Myopia.

Q.5: Explain how X-rays can be used in medicine. What are the limitations of conventional X-rays and how they can be overcome?

Q.6: What is ionizing radiation and how does it damage living organisms? What measures are taken to re- duce exposure to X-rays in hospital?

Q.7: When we enter the dark room, why we have to wait for sometime to see the things in the room.

Q.8: Describe the main features of eye and show how it forms images.

Q.9: Barium sulfate is used to outline organs. Explain.

Q.10: Irradiation by UV rays in case of neonatal jaundice.

Q.11: Lens of the eye and accommodation.

Q.12: Causes of blackout of vision at high angular acceleration.

■ BIBLIOGRAPHY

1. Cassidy D, Holton G, Rutherford J. Understanding Physics. Birkhäuser, 2002.
2. Hallo GH. Camera lenses: from box camera to digital. SPIE Press, 2006.
3. Hamarneh S. Review of Hakim Mohammed Said, Ibn al-Haitham, Isis, 1972; 63 (1): 119.
4. InformedHealth.org [Internet]. Cologne, Germany: Institute for Quality and Efficiency in Health Care (IQWiG); 2006-. Presbyopia: Overview. [Updated 2020 Jun 4]. Available from: https://www.ncbi.nlm.nih.gov/books/NBK423833/
5. Kalumuck KE. Human body explorations: hands-on investigations of what makes us tick. Kendall Hunt, 2000.
6. Kumar N. Comprehensive Physics XII. Laxmi Publications, 2008.
7. Longair, Malcolm. Theoretical Concepts in Physics, 2003: 87.
8. MacKay RJ, Oldford RW. "Scientific Method, Statistical Method and the Speed of Light", Statistical Science, August 2000, 15 (3): 254–78.
9. Majumdar S, Tripathy K. Hyperopia. [Updated 2022 Feb 21]. In: StatPearls [Internet]. Treasure Island (FL): StatPearls Publishing; 2022 Jan-. Available from: https://www.ncbi.nlm.nih.gov/books/NBK560716/
10. Nichols EF, Hull GF. The Pressure due to Radiation, The Astrophysical Journal, 1903;17 (5):315–51.
11. Ptolemy, Smith AM. Ptolemy's Theory of Visual Perception: An English Translation of the Optics with Introduction and Commentary. Diane Publishing, 1996.
12. Rashed, Roshdi. "The Celestial Kinematics of Ibn al-Haytham", Arabic Sciences and Philosophy. Cambridge University Press, 2007.
13. Singh P, Tripathy K. Presbyopia. [Updated 2022 Feb 21]. In: StatPearls [Internet]. Treasure Island (FL): StatPearls Publishing; 2022 Jan-. Available from: https://www.ncbi.nlm.nih.gov/books/NBK560568/
14. Verma RL. Al-Hazen: father of modern optics, 1969.
15. Vyasa, Krishna-Dwai. The Mahabharata of Krishna-Dwaipayana Vyasa 1st Book Adi Parva, The Echo Library, 2000.

CHAPTER 7

Pressure and Fluid Mechanics

Navjot Kaur, Shiv Kumar Mudgal

CHAPTER OUTLINE
- Importance of Pressure in the Human Body
- Atmospheric Pressure
- Applications of Atmospheric Pressure
- Hydrostatic Pressure
- Applications of Pascal's Law
- Pressure in Flowing Fluids
- Osmotic Pressure
- Applications of the Osmotic Pressure
- Measurement of Pressures
- Applications of these Principles in Nursing

■ INTRODUCTION

In day-to-day life, we use the word pressure in a number of different contexts. Students feel the pressure of work during examination days. Many a time we talk of political pressure. When the water coming out of our taps has low-speed, we say that water pressure is low. The steam pressure is used to cook food. Air pressure in car tyres permits safe driving. The weather man tells us the atmospheric pressure and the doctor measures our blood pressure. In physics, like work, pressure has a definite meaning. It is defined as follows:

"Pressure is the force on a unit surface area".

If the force F is acting on a surface of area A, the pressure P is given by:

$$P \frac{F}{A}$$

- ❖ The pressure exerted by fluids is called fluid pressure.
- ❖ The SI unit of pressure is called Pascal and is denoted by the symbol 'Pa'.

- Pressure has no fixed direction and is therefore a scalar quantity.
  - You probably know that atmospheric pressure is about 10^5 Pa. In medical practice, the most common method of indicating pressure is by the height of a column of mercury. The pressure of a column of liquid can be calculated using the relation:
  $$P = hdg$$
  - Where 'd' is the density of the liquid, 'g' is the acceleration due to gravity and 'h' is the height of the liquid column.

■ IMPORTANCE OF PRESSURE IN THE HUMAN BODY

Knowledge of pressure is needed to understand the functioning of the human body. Body cavities and organs are affected by pressure both in health and in disease. For example:
- Normal breathing depends partially on differences in intrapleural and intrapulmonic pressures and changes in pressure may produce respiratory distress.
- The effectiveness of treatments such as enemas and other irrigations depends on pressure.
- Many body functions depend on fluid pressure. For example, the heart pumps blood through the arteries at quite high-pressure (100–140 mm Hg). The returning venous blood is at quite low-pressure and has to be helped to go from the legs to the heart. Some typical values of the fluid pressures in the body are given in **Table 7.1**.

Table 7.1: Typical pressure in a normal and healthy human body.

Body/organ pressure	The typical value of pressure (in mm Hg)
Arterial blood pressure	
Maximum	100–140
Minimum	60–90
Venous blood pressure	3–7
Intrathoracic pressure (between lung and chest wall)	10
Capillary blood pressure	
Arterial end	30
Venous end	10
Middle ear pressure	<1
Urinary bladder	<2
Eye pressure—aqueous humor	20
Cerebrospinal fluid pressure in brain	5-12
Gastrointestinal pressure	10-20

■ ATMOSPHERIC PRESSURE

The air around us has weight, and it presses against everything it touches, that pressure is called atmospheric pressure, or air pressure. It is the force exerted on a surface by the air above, it as gravity pulls it to Earth. Atmospheric pressure drops as altitude increases.

As the pressure decreases, the amount of oxygen available to breathe also decreases. At very high altitudes, atmospheric pressure and available oxygen get so low that people can become sick and even die.

The atmospheric pressure was first measured by Torricelli nearly three centuries ago following some observations of the Duke of Tuscany (Italy). The Duke got a deep well dug and found that the suction pumps available at that time failed to lift water to a height of more than about 34 feet (10 m). To discover the answer to this curious phenomenon, Torricelli took a long glass tube open at one end and filled it with mercury. He closed the open end of the tube with his finger and inverted it into a vessel containing mercury. When he removed his finger, he observed that the level of mercury dropped to a certain height, leaving an empty space at the top. This empty space is known as the Torricellian vacuum **(Fig. 7.1)**.

The length of the column of mercury was found to be nearly 30 feet, i.e., 76 cm. It was also found that the level of mercury in the tube is independent of its cross-section as well as its inclination.

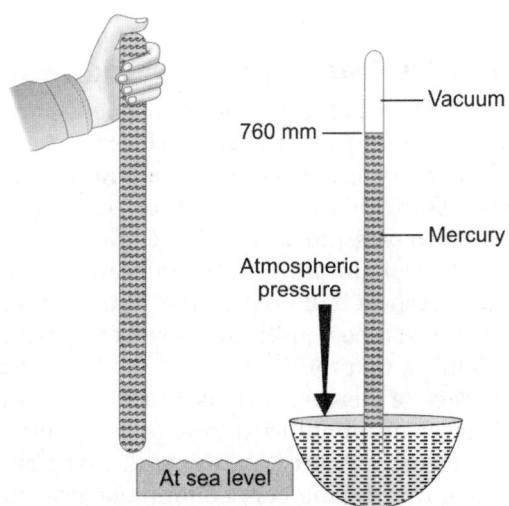

Fig. 7.1: Torricelli experiment.

By performing this experiment, Torricelli showed that the height of a liquid column cannot rise beyond a certain height because, it is experimentally determined by the atmospheric pressure. Thus, the water from the well got dug by the Duke of Tuscany did not rise beyond on and mercury in Torricelli's experiment did not rise beyond 76 cm. In this way, Torricelli was able to clear the confusion of the Duke of Tuscany.

Above the earth's surface, there is a vast quantity of air which is a mixture of many gases, is termed as atmosphere. The weight of the atmosphere exerts a force on the surface of every object on or near the surface of the earth. At sea level, this force produces a pressure of 14.7 lb/in^2. Torricelli found that at sea level the atmospheric pressure is sufficient to maintain the mercury column at 76 cm above the surface of the mercury in the container. Atmospheric pressure is sometimes expressed in terms of cm of mercury as 76 cm Hg or 760 mm Hg. This is equivalent to a pressure of 14.7 lb/in^2.

Mountain climbers use bottled oxygen when they ascend very high peaks. They also take time to get used to the altitude because quickly moving from higher pressure to lower pressure can cause decompression sickness. Decompression sickness also called "the bends", is also a problem for scuba divers who come to the surface too quickly. Aircraft create artificial pressure in the cabin so passengers remain comfortable while flying.

Atmospheric pressure is an indicator of weather. When a low-pressure system moves into an area, it usually leads to cloudiness, wind, and precipitation. High-pressure systems usually lead to fair, calm weather.

The Instrument for Measuring Atmospheric Pressure

An instrument used for measuring the atmospheric pressure is called a barometer. It is made up of a glass tube closed at one end, and it is filled up with mercury and inverted into a bowl of mercury. When atmospheric pressure increases, the level of the mercury column in the tube rises, when pressure decreases the level of the column falls.

Let us further elaborate on the inferences, of Torricelli's experiment with respect to fluid pressure. You can visualize this as follows: When a glass tube is inverted in a vessel containing mercury, Pascal's law implies that the pressure exerted by the atmosphere on the free surface of mercury is transmitted equally over its entire volume. This gives us an upthrust base of the inverted glass tube and pushes mercury upwards. As a result, mercury rises in the tube till the weight of the mercury column balances the up-thrust.

Therefore, the height of this column is equivalent to the pressure of the atmosphere on the free surface of the mercury in the vessel. If the height of the mercury column in the tube above the free surface of the mercury in the container is 'h' and the density of mercury is 'd', then the atmospheric pressure is given by:

$$P = hdg$$

Thus, the normal atmospheric pressure is written as 760 mm Hg (or 76 cm Hg). If the pressure is below 760 mm Hg, it is said to be sub-atmospheric (that is, less than atmospheric pressure).

You may ask: Can we create sub-atmospheric pressure? Yes; if all gases are confined in a container could be recovered from it so that a perfect vacuum is created, then pressure becomes zero. However, practically it is not possible to create a perfect vacuum, and only a partial vacuum can be created. These partial vacuums give rise to a sub-atmospheric pressure. Since fluids (liquids and gases) flow from points of higher pressure to those of lower pressure, fluids above atmospheric pressure will flow into a vessel that is at sub-atmospheric pressure.

Applications of Atmospheric Pressure

- Suction is a process by which a region having sub-atmospheric pressure can be created. It is employed during surgical operation for the removal of blood and serosanguineous fluids from the region of the human body being operated.
- Many kinds of aspirators in the hospital wards work on the application of controlled suction.
- Water-seal drainage used after thoracic operations works on controlled suction and gravity.
- Suction apparatus for drainage in the postoperation treatment of patients with alimentary tract disorders are commonly observed in surgical wards.
- Tidal drainage by means of gravity flow and siphonage initiates the natural physiological process of the urinary bladder.
- Pressure greater than atmospheric pressure is applied by numerous mechanical devices to alleviate disturbing pulmonary functions (Birds Respirator Oxygen Tent).
- Pumps are dependent on their functioning on atmospheric pressure. A pump operates on the principle of pressure gradients, i.e., that fluids move from places of greater to those of lesser pressure.
- In hospitals, pumps can be used to fill air rings and air mattresses or to remove fluids from body cavities.

- The human heart operates in many ways like a pump. The right and left ventricles of the heart function like two synchronized pumps. They keep the flow of blood streaming continuously in one direction. The right ventricle pumps venous blood to the lungs. At the same time, the left ventricle pumps oxygenated blood to the tissues of the body. The ventricles are equipped with two sets of valves, the atrioventricular valve, and the semilunar valves. As the ventricles fill, the pressure within them increases. When the ventricles contract, the increased pressure closed the atrioventricular valves and opens the semilunar valves.
- **Siphon:** It is a device made of glass or rubber tubing with one short and long arm. It is used to move a liquid, the surface of which is exposed to the atmosphere, from a higher to a lower level. The siphon is so arranged that the shorter arm is placed in the liquid to be emptied and the longer arm is placed in a container at a lower level **(Fig. 7.2)**. The decompression apparatus for emptying the urinary bladder and the munro tidal drainage apparatus operate partially by siphon. A siphon is also the basis of action in gastric lavage. A rubber tube is passed into the stomach. After the stomach is filled with fluid, the funnel and tube are turned downward to form the long arm of the siphon. When there is no air in the system fluid will flow out of the stomach.

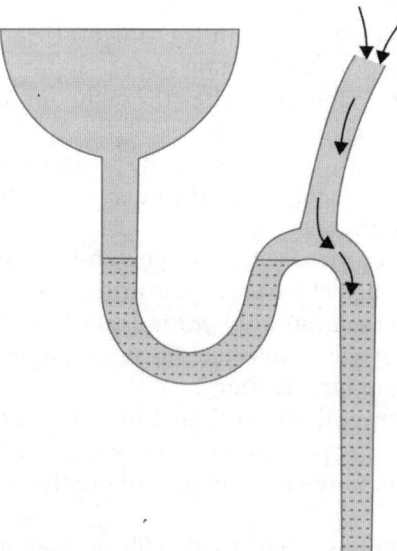

Fig. 7. 2: Siphon.

■ HYDROSTATIC PRESSURE

Hydrostatic pressure refers to the pressure that is exerted, due to the force of gravity, by a fluid at equilibrium at any particular point of time. Furthermore, hydrostatic pressure is proportional to the depth whose measurement takes place from the surface as the increase in weight of the fluid happens. Moreover, this increase in weight happens when a downward force is applied.

This very important property of all fluids (gases and liquids) was discovered by Pascal. He observed that when pressure is applied to a confined fluid, it is transmitted uniformly throughout its volume. He stated this observation in the form of a law, which is known as Pascal's law. We may state it as:

"Any change of pressure applied at any point in an enclosed fluid at rest is transmitted undiminished and uniformly to all its parts transpose".

Liquids that are enclosed in a vessel produce pressure by virtue of their weight. The pressure at any point below the surface is proportional to the weight of the column of liquid above that point. If a substance is twice as heavy as water, the pressure will be doubled. The pressure at any point below the surface can be determined by knowing the height of the liquid column and the density of the liquid, i.e.

$$P = hdg$$

Where,
   P = pressure
   h = height
   d = density
   g = acceleration due to gravity (is constant for a particular place)

For example:
Fluid in an enema container or in irrigating equipment exerts pressure by virtue of the weight of the column of fluid above the point of exit of the fluid. The greater the column of fluid is an enema container the greater the pressure at the level where it enters the body. The same principle applies to intravenous infusions and other parenteral fluids.

Applications of Pascal's Law

Pascal's law has been put to a variety of uses in day-to-day life as well as healthcare practices.
- ❖ In medicine, the use of water-mattress and air-rings work on the same principle. These mattresses are used to prevent bedsores in bedridden patients.

- The amniotic sac enclosing the fetus in the uterus is filled with amniotic fluid, which is a confined fluid and serves as a protection to the fetus. Any pressure exerted against the abdominal wall will be transmitted to the amniotic fluid to all surfaces of the fetus. To avoid unequal pressure, which may cause fetal deformity, the patient is usually cautioned against wearing tight clothing during pregnancy.
- Lumbar puncture and spinal fluid flow test to locate the blockage in the flow of CSF is also based on this principle only.
- In sphygmomanometer, the mercury manometer operates on the principle of Pascal's law. The flow of blood in the artery is occluded by the pressure of the enclosed air in the airtight cuff. The pressure supports a column of mercury in the manometer. When the air in the cuff is released slowly, the blood just begins to flow again; the pressure is measured by the height of this mercury column **(Fig. 7.3A)**.
- Medicine droppers and rubber bulb syringes enclose a fluid also work on the principle of Pascal's law. Pressure applied against the rubber bulb is transmitted to the enclosed liquid and caused it to flow from the open end of the dropper or syringe **(Fig. 7.3B)**.
- Hydraulic brakes, are used in aircraft, automobiles, and trucks.
- The hydraulic press, is used to compress metal sheets, wool, or bales of cotton.
- Hydraulic carjacks, these are collectively referred to as hydraulic machines. A hydraulic jack is used to lift heavy vehicles in an automobile workshop. A force is applied on the piston of a smaller area of cross-section. The piston is gradually pushed inwards and the automobile moves upwardly.

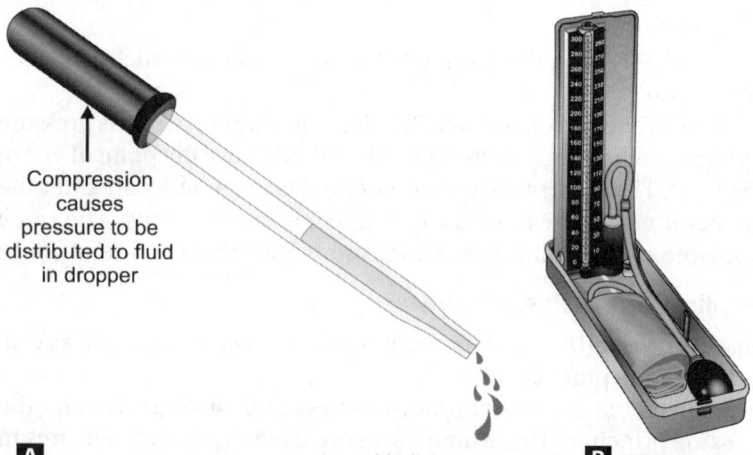

A Compression causes pressure to be distributed to fluid in dropper

Medicine comes out **B** BP apparatus

Figs. 7.3A and B: Working applications of Pascal's law.

- The dentist's chair also works on the same principle. The seat of the chair is placed over the larger piston and the smaller piston is operated by a foot pedal.
- Heavy lids of some sterilizers are lifted by using the same principle.
- The latest technology hospital beds also work on the sample principle, where the position of the patient can be changed very easily by a small piston operated by hand or foot.

■ PRESSURE IN FLOWING FLUIDS

You now know that some of the observed properties of fluids at rest can be understood in terms of simple concepts like pressure, density, and Pascal's law. You can now ask: What happens when fluids are in motion? The knowledge of the dynamics of the flowing fluid is important to understand the flow of blood in the circulatory system, in the preparation and administration of blood transfusions, intravenous infusions, etc.

An important requirement for the flow of fluids in a system is pressure gradient, i.e., difference in pressures at the ends of the system:

"Fluid flows from a region of higher pressure to that of lower pressure".

Breathing (that is, the flow of air in and out of the human body) is possible due to pressure differences. Further, the flow rate, i.e., volume of liquid flowing out per second, through a straight tube of the uniform cross-section is directly proportional to the pressure gradient across it. During internal hemorrhage, blood flows out of the blood vessel, and the pressure drops within the circulatory system.

Other factors being equal, the flow of fluid through an orifice depends on:
- **Area of the orifice:** The larger the orifice, the greater is the fluid flow.
- **The pressure gradient:** The greater the pressure gradient; the greater is the rate of flow.

However, when a fluid flows through a pipe of varying cross-section, irregular motion or turbulent flow occurs and the speed of flow in a pipe increases at a constriction. This suggests a connection between high blood pressure and the thickening of arteries. For flowing the same amount of blood in a narrowed artery, more pressure is required. Normally, the flow of blood in blood vessels of our body is laminar (uniform).

But when blood vessels develop roughened walls or linings, or there is some bulging, turbulent flow of blood may rupture the delicate platelets in the blood and initiate the formation of blood clots in the vessel or bloodstream. Such internal hemorrhages possess a serious threat to life.

Some of the important relations among various physical parameters of fluids are known as different laws given below:

- ❖ ***Boyle's law*** states that the volume of a gas varies inversely with the pressure if the temperature is constant. This law is the basis of the working of a sphygmomanometer (BP apparatus).
- ❖ ***Charles's law*** states that the pressure of a gas is directly proportional to its temperature if the volume is kept constant. Many of the pressure cookers and autoclave machines work on these principles.
- ❖ ***Dalton's law*** states that in a gas mixture, the pressure exerted by each individual gas in space is independent of the pressures of other gases in the mixture. This principle is used while giving general anesthesia.

■ OSMOTIC PRESSURE

- ❖ Osmosis is the process by which solvent moves from a region of lesser concentration of solutes to a higher concentration of solutes through a semipermeable membrane.
- ❖ It may be defined as the equivalent of the external pressure that must be applied to a solution in order to prevent the passage of the solvent into it through a perfect semi-permeable membrane.
- ❖ The osmotic pressure of a solution is proportional to the concentration of the solute particles that cannot cross the membrane. The higher the solute concentration, the higher the solution's osmotic pressure.
- ❖ In the case of substances that ionize, the osmotic pressure that would be expected from the concentration alone will actually be greater because of a larger number of particles per molecule than one.
- ❖ Osmotic pressure is the pressure caused by water at different concentrations due to the dilution of water by dissolved molecules (solute), notably salts and nutrients.

For example:

- ❖ Sodium chloride solution will contain two particles, one sodium ion, and one chloride ion, for each molecule of sodium chloride. Osmotic pressure from substances such as sodium chloride that are strong electrolytes (i.e., ionize to a great extent) will be higher

than that produced by substances that ionize weakly or not at all, other things being equal. In addition, the size of the molecules in the solution has an effect on osmotic pressure.
- ❖ Osmotic pressure is closely related to some other properties of solutions, the colligative properties. These include the freezing point depression, the boiling point elevation, and the vapor pressure depression, all caused by dissolving solutes in a solution.

Measuring Osmotic Pressure

Osmotic pressure can be measured in various ways which are described below: 1. Mechanical Methods, 2. Biological Methods, 3. Physical Methods.

Mechanical Methods

By Putting Weights

The simplest way is to apply adequate pressure (i.e., weight) upon the stronger solution to prevent any rise of volume. That pressure, which is just needed to stop the increase of volume of a particular solution is the measure of its OP. If a piston is used to apply more pressure to the fluid in the right arm, with enough pressure, the volume of pressure in each arm could be restored to the starting volume and the concentration of the solute in the right arm would be the same as it was in the beginning. The amount of pressure needed to restore the starting condition equals the osmotic pressure **(Fig. 7.4).**

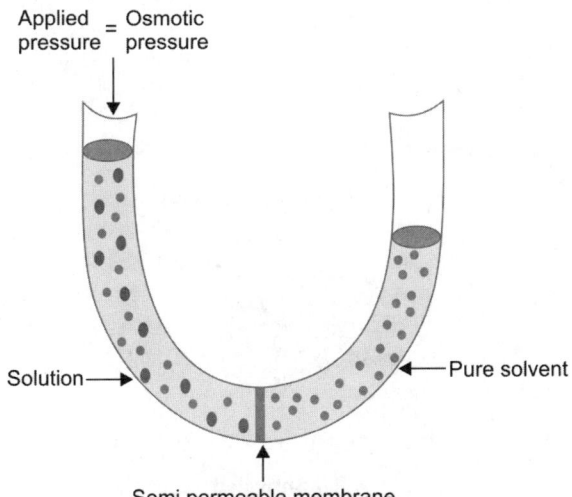

Fig. 7.4: Measurement of osmotic pressure.

By a Manometer

The same thing can be done by connecting the apparatus with a suitable manometer, in which the pressure will gradually rise till it equalizes with the osmotic pressure of the solution, at which point further rise will stop (Pfeffer's method).

Biological Methods

Hamburger's Red Corpuscle Method:

Red cells are kept in the unknown solution for some time, after which the cell volume is noted. If the cell volume is reduced, the solution is hypertonic than plasma (hence, water has been drawn out), if the cells swell up, the solution is hypotonic (so that water has entered), and if no change—the solution is isotonic, if sufficiently hypotonic the red cells will gradually swell up and ultimately burst (Hemolysis) (**Fig. 7.5**).

Physical Methods

By noting depression of freezing point. Higher the concentration, lower will be the freezing point, and therefore higher will be the osmotic pressure.

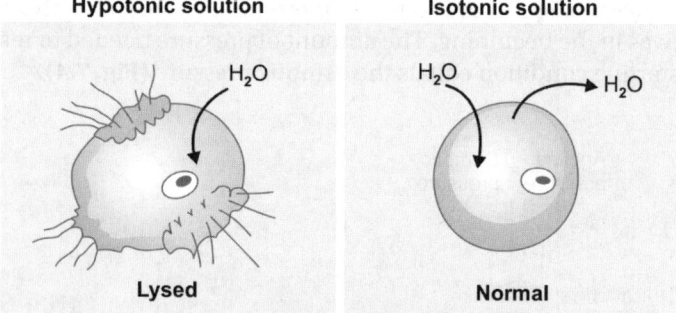

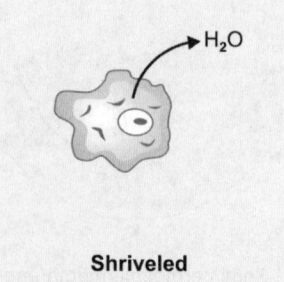

Fig. 7.5: Fate of RBC in different solution.

By Noting the Vapor Tension
Higher the concentration, lower will be the rate of evaporation from the solution and higher the osmotic pressure.

Hill's Method
Using thermopile; the higher the rate of evaporation more will be the fall of temperature and less will be the osmotic pressure. Comparison is made with a solution of known osmotic pressure.

Burger's Capillary Glass Tube Method
Alternate drops of known and unknown solutions separated by air bubbles are drawn in a standard capillary glass tube and after some time the edges of the solutions are noted. The edges will shift according to the rate of evaporation. From these data, Osmotic Pressure can be calculated.

Applications of the Osmotic Pressure

- Blood albumin helps to maintain the colloidal pressure of the blood. At the capillaries, this pressure is effective in maintaining the normal fluid content of the blood. If a patient loses blood albumin which may happen in nephrosis the colloidal osmotic pressure will drop and fluid remains in the tissues. This results in edema.
- Sometimes infusion of a hypertonic solution is useful to treat patients who have cerebral edema, and excess interstitial fluid in the brain like mannitol. It relieves such fluid overload by causing osmosis of water from the interstitial fluid into the blood. Then the kidneys excrete excess water from the blood into the urine.
- Administration of hypotonic solutions either IV or oral, can be used to treat people who are dehydrated. The water in the hypotonic solution moves from the blood into the interstitial fluid and then into the body cells to rehydrate them.
- In dialysis along with diffusion, osmosis also works.

■ MEASUREMENT OF PRESSURES

Arterial Pressure

The cardiovascular system has three types of pressures: hemodynamic, kinetic energy, and hydrostatic. Hemodynamic pressure is the energy imparted to the blood by the contraction of the left ventricle. This type of pressure is preserved by the elastic properties of the arterial system. Kinetic energy is the energy associated with motion and affects the pressure measured during direct arterial BP monitoring. Fluid density and gravity contribute to hydrostatic pressure, which is the pressure a column of fluid exerts on the container's wall. For example, in a column of fluid, the pressure at a given level in the container is proportional to the height of the fluid column above that level. The pressure is highest at the bottom of the column. In the vascular system, hydrostatic pressure is proportional to the height of the column of blood between the heart and the peripheral vasculature. In a standing person, the pressure in the leg is higher than the pressure in the arm by the difference in hydrostatic pressure. In summary, arterial blood pressure represents the force exerted by the blood per unit area on the arterial wall and is the sum of hemodynamic, kinetic, and hydrostatic pressure.

Measuring Arterial Pressure

The arterial pressure is measured using a sphygmomanometer (i.e., blood pressure cuff) on the upper arm, the systolic and diastolic pressures that are measured represent the pressure within the brachial artery, which is slightly different from the pressure found in the aorta or the pressure found in other distributing arteries. As the aortic pressure pulse travels down the aorta and into distributing arteries, there are characteristic changes in the systolic and diastolic pressures, as well as in the mean pressure. The systolic pressure rises and the diastolic pressure falls, therefore, the pulse pressure increases, as the pressure pulse travels away from the aorta. This occurs because of reflective waves from vessel branching, and from decreased arterial compliance (increased vessel stiffness) as the pressure pulse travels from the aorta into systemic arteries. There is only a small decline in mean arterial pressure as the pressure pulse travels down distributing arteries due to the relatively low resistance of large distributing arteries. Arterial blood pressure also can be measured by placing an intra-arterial catheter and directly attaching it to a monitor through a transducer.

Central Venous Pressure

Central venous pressure, which is a measure of pressure in the vena cava, can be used as an estimation of preload and right atrial pressure. Central venous pressure is often used as an assessment of hemodynamic status, particularly in the intensive care unit. The central venous pressure can be measured using a central venous catheter advanced via the internal jugular vein and placed in the superior vena cava near the right atrium.

Measuring Central Venous Pressure (CVP)

The CVP can be measured either manually using a manometer or electronically using a transducer. In either case, the CVP must be 'zeroed' at the level of the right atrium. This is usually taken to be the level of the 4th intercostal space in the midaxillary line while the patient is lying supine. Each measurement of CVP should be taken at this same zero position. Trends in the serial measurement of CVP are much more informative than single readings. However, if the CVP is measured at a different level each time, then this renders the trend in measurement inaccurate. CVP can be measured in two ways as described below:

- **Using the manometer:** A 3-way tap is used to connect the manometer to an intravenous drip set on one side, and via extension tubing filled with intravenous fluid, to the patient on the other. It is important to ensure that there are no air bubbles in the tubing, to avoid administering an air embolus to the patient. You should also check that the CVP catheter tubing is not kinked or blocked, that intravenous fluid can easily be flushed in and that blood can easily be aspirated from the line. The 3-way tap is then turned so that it is open to the fluid bag and the manometer but closed to the patient, allowing the manometer column to fill with fluid. It is important not to overfill the manometer, so preventing the cotton wool bung at the manometer tip from getting wet. Once the manometer has filled adequately the 3-way tap is turned again—this time, so it is open to the patient and the manometer, but closed to the fluid bag. The fluid level within the manometer column will fall to the level of the CVP, the value of which can be read on the manometer scale which is marked in centimeters, therefore giving a value for the CVP in centimeters of water (cm H_2O). The fluid level will continue to rise and fall slightly with respiration and the average reading should be recorded.
- **Using the transducer:** The transducer is fixed at the level of the right atrium and connected to the patient's CVP catheter via fluid-filled extension tubing. Similar care should be taken to avoid bubbles and kinks, etc. as mentioned above. The transducer is then 'zeroed' to atmospheric pressure by turning its 3-way tap so that it is open to the transducer and to the room air, but closed to the patient. The 3-way tap is then turned so that it is now closed to room air and open between the patient and the transducer. A continuous CVP reading, measured in mm Hg rather than cm H_2O, can be obtained.

Intraocular Pressure

Intraocular pressure (IOP) is the fluid pressure inside the eye. As pressure is a measure of force per area, IOP is a measurement involving the magnitude of the force exerted by the aqueous humor on the internal surface area of the anterior eye. Intraocular pressure is measured with a tonometer.

Tonometry is the measurement of tension or pressure within the eye. A tonometer is an instrument for measuring tension or pressure., Tonometry is the procedure, that eye care professionals perform to determine the intraocular pressure (IOP), the fluid pressure inside the eye. It is an important test in the evaluation of patients with glaucoma. Most tonometer's are calibrated to measure pressure in mm Hg.

Measuring Intraocular Pressure

There are three basic methods to measure intraocular pressure. A brief description of these methods are as follows:

- **Applanation method:** It measures the intraocular pressure either by a force required to flatten a constant area of the cornea (Goldmann tonometry) or by the area flattened by a constant force.
  - In applanation tonometry, a special calibrated disinfected probe attached to a slit lamp biomicroscope is used to flatten the central cornea by a fixed amount. Because the probe makes contact with the cornea, a topical anesthetic, such as oxybuprocaine, tetracaine, etc. is introduced onto the surface of the eye in the form of one or two eye drops. A yellow fluorescein dye is used in conjunction with a cobalt blue filter to aid the examiner in determining the IOP.
- **Dynamic contour tonometry:** Dynamic contour tonometry (DCT) is a novel method that uses the principle of contour matching instead of applanation.
- The pascal tonometer is currently the only commercial DCT tonometer available. It uses a miniature pressure sensor embedded within a tonometer tip contour matched to the shape of the cornea. The tonometer tip rests on the cornea with a constant appositional force of one gram. When the sensor is subjected to a change in pressure, the electrical resistance is altered and the pascal's computer calculates a change in pressure in concordance with the change in resistance.
- **Pneumatonometry:** A pneumatonometer utilizes a pneumatic sensor (consisting of a piston floating on an air bearing). It is touched to the anesthetized cornea. A precisely regulated flow of filtered air (from an internal air pump) enters the piston. A small (5 mm dia.) fenestrated membrane at the end of the piston reacts to both the force of the air blowing through it and to the force represented by the pressure behind the cornea, against which it

is being pressed. The precise balance between these two forces represents the precise intraocular pressure.

Intracranial Pressure

Intracranial pressure (ICP) is the pressure in the cranium and thus in the brain tissue and cerebrospinal fluid (CSF); this pressure is exerted on the brain's intracranial blood circulation vessels. ICP is maintained in a tight normal range dynamically, through the production and absorption of CSF and pulsates approximately 1 mm Hg in normal healthy adults. CSF pressure has been shown to be influenced by abrupt changes in intrathoracic pressure during coughing (intra-abdominal pressure), Valsalva maneuver, and communication with the vasculature (venous and arterial systems). ICP is measured in millimeters of mercury (mm Hg) and, at rest, is normally 7-15 mm Hg for a supine adult, and becomes negative (averaging –10 mm Hg) in the vertical position. Changes in ICP are attributed to volume changes in one or more of the constituents contained in the cranium.

Measuring Intracranial Pressure

There are two basic techniques or methods of measuring intracranial pressure.
- ❖ **Noninvasive methods**
  - Clinical deterioration in neurological status is widely considered a sign of increased ICP. Bradycardia, increased pulse pressure, and pupillary dilation are normally accepted as signs of increased ICP. The clinical monitoring is age-old and time tested.
  - Transcranial Doppler, tympanic membrane displacement, and ultrasound 'time of flight' techniques have been advocated. Several devices have been described for measuring ICP through open fontanel. Ladd fiber optic system has been used extracutaneously.
  - Manual feeling of the craniotomy flap or skull defect, if any, gives a clue.
- ❖ **Invasive methods**
  - Intraventricular monitoring remains one of the popular techniques, especially in patients with ventriculomegaly. The additional advantage is the potential for draining CSF therapeutically. Insertion of the ventricular catheter is not always simple and can cause hemorrhage and infection (5%).
  - Other most commonly used devices are the hollow screw and bolt devices, and the subdural catheter. Richmond screw and Becker bolt are used extradurally. A fluid-filled catheter in the

subdural space, connected to an arterial pressure monitoring system is cost-effective and serves the purpose adequately.
- The Ladd device is currently in wide use. It employs a fiberoptic system to detect the distortion of a tiny mirror within with balloon system. It can be used in the subdural, extradural, and even extracutaneously.
- A mechanically coupled surface monitoring device is the 'cardio search pneumatic sensor' used subdurally or extradurally. These systems are not widely used.
- Electronic devices (Camino & Galtesh design) are getting popular the world over. Intraparenchymal probes, the measured pressure may be compartmentalized and not necessarily representative of real ICP. In addition to ICP monitoring, modern intraparenchymal sensors help study the chemical environment of the site of pathology.
- Fully implantable devices are valuable in a small group that requires long-term ICP monitoring for brain tumors, hydrocephalus, or other chronic brain diseases. Common intracranial pressure tele sensor can be implanted as a part of the shunt system. Ommaya reservoir is an alternative that can be punctured and CSF pressure readings are obtained.
- Lumbar puncture and measurement of CSF pressure for obvious reasons are not recommended.

■ APPLICATIONS OF THESE PRESSURES IN NURSING

Applications of different types of pressures in healthcare practices and nursing procedures are discussed with the description of each type of pressure. Therefore, you can refer to the application of different pressures as discussed individually in the chapter.

■ QUESTIONS

Q.1: State Pascal's law. Give two examples of its application in the human body.
Q.2: How can we create sub-atmospheric pressure? Give two applications from the nursing procedure.
Q.3: Force acting on the unit surface is called as...............
Q.4: Mouth to mouth respiration in respiratory distress. Explain.
Q.5: What is pressure, osmotic diuresis, and diffusion?
Q.6: What are the physiological functions of the human body that depend upon the osmotic pressure and dialysis for their normal function?
Q.7: Occurrence of edema in nephrosis. Discuss.
Q.8: Why a chronic bedridden patient is advised to use an air-mattress instead of an ordinary mattress?

Q.9: Heart as a double compression pump. Discuss.
Q.10: Positive pressure is applied to patients with pulmonary edema. Discuss.
Q.11: When the normal breathing stops in a drowsed person, artificial respiration helps to restore it?
Q.12: Factors affecting pressure and the two pressures in the human body. Explain.

■ BIBLIOGRAPHY

1. Atkins P, J de Paula. Elements of Physical Chemistry, Fourth edition, WH. Freeman, 2006.
2. Cotterill RMJ. Biophysics: An Introduction. Wiley, 2002.
3. Dogonadze RR, Urushadze ZD. "Semi-Classical Method of Calculation of Rates of Chemical Reactions Proceeding in Polar Liquids". J Electroanal Chem, 1971; 32: 235-45.
4. Giancoli, Douglas G. Physics: Principles with applications. Upper Saddle River, NJ: Pearson Education, 2004.
5. Hobbie RK, Roth BJ. International Physics for Medicine and Biology (Fourth edition). Springer, 2006.
6. Perutz MF. Proteins and Nucleic Acids: Structure and Function. Amsterdam: Elsevier, 1962.
7. Roland G. Biophysics: An Introduction (Corrected edition). Springer, 2004: 11-23.
8. Sneppen K, Zocchi G. Physics in Molecular Biology, First edition. Cambridge University Press, 2005:10-17.
9. Volkenshtein MV, Dogonadze RR, Madumarov AK. Theory of Enzyme Catalysis. Molekuliarnaya Biologia (Moscow)1972; 6: 431-39 (In Russian, English summary).
10. Darwish A, Lui F. Physiology, Colloid Osmotic Pressure. [Updated 2021 Oct 1]. In: StatPearls [Internet]. Treasure Island (FL): StatPearls Publishing; 2022 Jan. Available from: https://www.ncbi.nlm.nih.gov/books/NBK541067/
11. Joseph Feher. Osmosis and Osmotic Pressure. Quantitative Human Physiology (Second Edition) Academic Press, 2017 Pages 182-198. Available from https://doi.org/10.1016/B978-0-12-800883-6.00017-3.
12. Shah P, Louis MA. Physiology, Central Venous Pressure. [Updated 2021 Sep 14]. In: StatPearls [Internet]. Treasure Island (FL): StatPearls Publishing; 2022 Jan. Available from: https://www.ncbi.nlm.nih.gov/books/NBK519493/
13. Machiele R, Motlagh M, Patel BCc. Intraocular Pressure. [Updated 2021 Jul 31]. In: StatPearls [Internet]. Treasure Island (FL): StatPearls Publishing; 2022 Jan. Available from: https://www.ncbi.nlm.nih.gov/books/NBK532237/

CHAPTER 8

Sound Waves

Rakhi Gaur, Navjot Kaur

CHAPTER OUTLINE
- Mechanism of Propagation of Waves
- Types of Waves
- Types of Wave Motion
- Sound Waves
- Some Important Terms Connected with Wave Motion
- Wave Phenomenon
- Characteristics of Sound
- Vocalization and Hearing
- Doppler Effect
- Applications
- Noise Pollution and its Prevention

■ INTRODUCTION

You must have seen that when we throw a piece of stone into the water in a pond, we observe ripples traveling on the surface of the water in concentric circles of ever-increasing radius, till they strike the boundary of the pond. When we put a piece of cork on the surface of this water, we observe that the cork piece moves up and down as the wave passes, but the piece does not travel along with the waves. Thus, the particles of the medium certainly oscillate about their mean position, but their displacement away from their mean position is not there. The water waves carry energy but there is no transfer of water. So, wave motion is the propagation of disturbances—that is, deviations from a state of rest or equilibrium—from place to place in a regular and organized way. Most familiar are surface waves on water, but both sound and light travel as wavelike disturbances and the motion of all subatomic particles exhibits wavelike properties.

So we can define, "wave motion as a kind of disturbance which travels through a material medium (having property of elasticity and inertia) or account of repeated periodic vibrations of the particles of medium about their mean position, the disturbance being handed on from one particle to the adjoining particle and so on, without any met transport of the medium".

The central feature of wave motion is "Energy is transferred over a distance but the matter is not".

■ MECHANISM OF PROPAGATION OF WAVES

Let us look at some of the important terms before understanding the mechanism of propagation of waves.

❖ **Kinetic energy:** It is the energy associated with motion.
$$KE = \tfrac{1}{2} mv^2$$

❖ **Potential energy:** It is stored energy and depends on an object's position
$$PE = mgh$$

- *Inertia:* It is the property by which particles can store energy and overshoot their position.
- *Elasticity:* It is the property by which particles can return to their mean position, after having been disturbed.

'XY' represents the horizontal surface of the water when a stone hits a particle of water at 'O', the particle moves down to 'A' **(Fig. 8.1)**. During the motion of particles from 'O' to 'A', a restoring force develops on account of the elasticity of the water. Work done

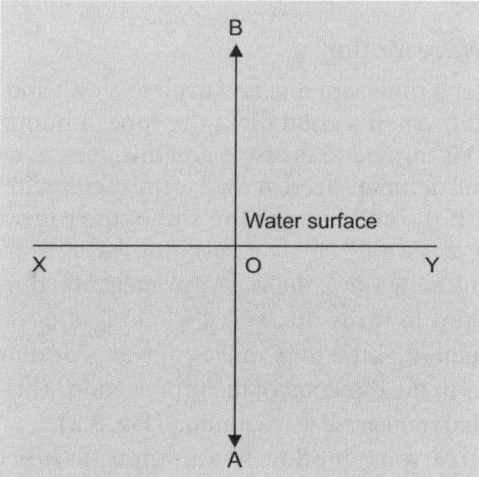

Fig. 8.1: Mechanism of propagation of waves.

against the restoring force while the particle moved from 'O' to 'A' is stored in the particle at 'A' in form of potential energy. From 'A', the particle moves towards 'O', under the action of restoring force. The potential energy of the particle is converted into kinetic energy at 'O'. On account of inertia, therefore the particle cannot stop at 'O'. It overshoots its mean position 'O' and goes over to B, the particle then moves back to 'O', under the action of restoring force again and so on. Thus, the particle of water at 'O' executes periodic vibrations due to elasticity and inertia.

This disturbance is communicated to the adjoining particles which also start vibrating simply harmonically about their mean positions. Hence, wave motion travels on and on at the water surface.

■ TYPES OF WAVES

- ❖ **Elastic waves or mechanical waves:** Waves that can be produced or propagated only in a material medium are called elastic waves or mechanical waves. For example, waves on the water surface, sound waves, etc.
- ❖ **Electromagnetic waves or non-mechanical waves:** The waves which can pass even through vacuum; for example, light waves from the sun, radiowaves, microwaves, X-rays, etc.

■ TYPES OF WAVE MOTION

The wave motion is primarily classified into two broad categories, i.e., transverse wave motion and longitudinal wave motion. The details are given below:

Transverse Wave Motion

Let us consider a rope with one end fixed to a wall and another end held by a child. When a child flicks the rope, a bump (technically called 'pulse') is formed in the rope and this pulse travels along the rope with some definite speed. A rope is the medium through which pulse travels. If the child moves the end of the rope up and down continuously, this would create a pulsating wave.

For this pulsating wave, the wave's propagation direction is from the child's hand towards the wall, i.e., along the rope, and each disturbing element of the rope moves upwards or downwards, i.e., perpendicular to the direction of the propagation. This kind of wave motion is called transverse wave motion **(Fig. 8.2)**.

A transverse wave motion is a motion in which individual particles of the medium execute simple harmonic motion about

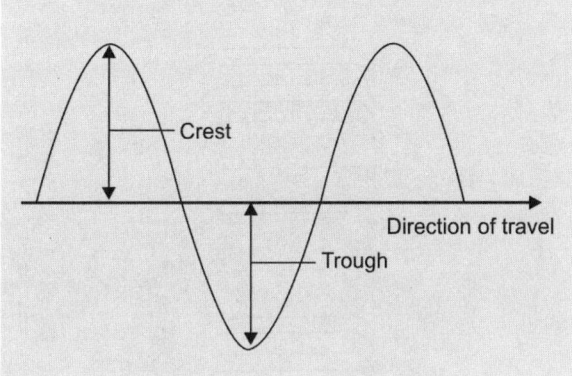

Fig. 8.2: Transverse wave motion.

their mean position in a direction perpendicular to the direction of propagation of wave motion. For example, movement of rope or string as described above.

* A transverse wave travels through a medium in the form of crests and troughs.
* The crest is a portion of the medium, which is raised temporarily above the normal position of the rest of the particles of the medium when a transverse wave passes through it.
* A trough is a portion of the medium, which is depressed temporarily below the normal position of the rest of the particles of the medium when a transverse wave passes through it.

Another example of transverse wave is a light wave. In light waves, electric and magnetic fields move perpendicular to the direction of propagation of light.

Longitudinal Wave Motion or Pressure Wave

A longitudinal wave motion is that wave motion in which individual particles of the medium execute simple harmonic motion about their mean position along the same direction along which the wave is propagated, for example, sound waves travel through the air in the form of longitudinal waves **(Fig. 8.3)**.

A longitudinal wave travels through a medium in the form of compressions or condensations (C) and rarefactions (R).

* **A compression:** It is a region of the medium in which particles are comprised, i.e., particles come closer (distance between the articles becomes less than the normal distance between them). Thus, there is a temporary decrease in volume and a consequent increase in the density of the medium in the region of compression.

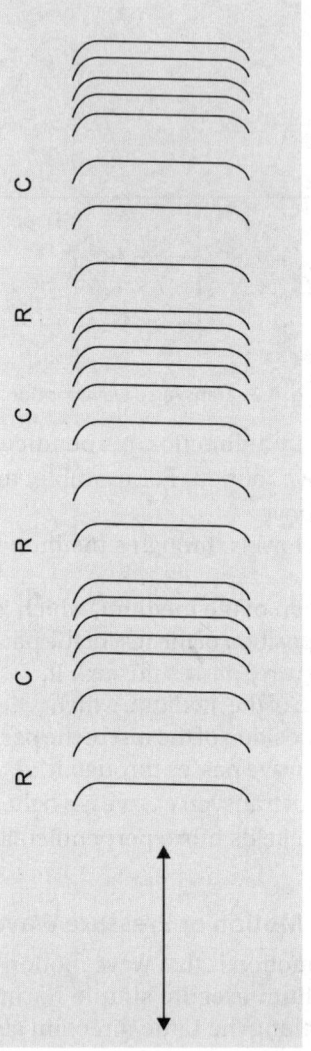

Fig. 8.3: Longitudinal wave motion.

- **A rarefaction:** It is a region of the medium in which particles are rarefied, i.e., particles get farther apart than they normally are. Thus, there is a temporary increase in volume and a consequent decrease in the density of the medium in the region of rarefaction.

A mechanical wave shall be transverse or longitudinal depending on:
- Nature of the medium.
- Mode of excitation of vibration

Example: In solid, mechanical waves can be either transverse or longitudinal. In strings, mechanical waves are always transverse. In liquids and gases, mechanical waves are generally longitudinal.

Though, all the waves cannot be characterized as longitudinal or transverse waves. For example, when a steady surface of the water is disturbed, waves are produced on the surface. Water particles move in a circular or elliptical fashion when a wave passes through them. An elliptical motion has both components, i.e., along and perpendicular to the wave motion.

■ SOUND WAVES

When we listen to a guitar or sitar sound, no material particle is ejected from the guitar or sitar and falls on our ears. It is just a disturbance in the part of the air close to the sitar. Energy is transferred to these air particles by pushing or strumming sitar wires. The disturbed air particles exert force on the next layer. In this way, the disturbance proceeds in medium (here air), and finally the air near our ear gets disturbed.

Hearing is one of the primary sensations. The physical cause that produces the sensation of hearing is the vibration of the source, e.g., when we listen to a sitar recital, the sitar wire vibrates. Sound is derived from objects that vibrate producing pressure variations in a sound-transmitting medium, such as air. A pressure wave is propagated outward from the vibrating source. When the pressure wave encounters another object, the vibration can be imparted to that object and the pressure wave will propagate in the medium of the object. The sound wave may also be reflected from the object or it may diffract around the object. Thus, a sound wave propagating outward from a vibrating object can reach the eardrum of a listener causing the eardrum to vibrate and initiate the process of hearing. Our ear is sensitive only to those vibrations whose frequency lies between 20 and 20,000 Hz. This frequency range is called the audible range.

"A vibration whose frequency is greater than 20,000 Hz is called ultrasonic vibration. The sound waves which have a frequency less than the audible range are called infrasonic waves. These cannot be heard by the human ear".

The velocity of sound in air at room temperature and normal pressure is roughly 332 ms^{-1} which is approximately 1200 kmh^{-1}. This is much greater than the speed of the fastest car. That is why the horn

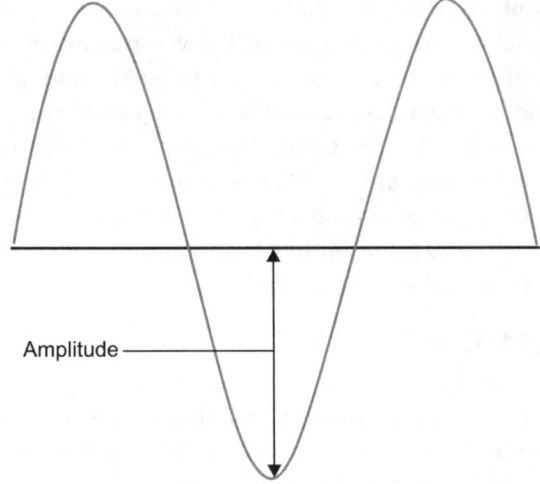

Fig. 8.4: Amplitude.

of a motor car approaching us is heard much before the car reaches us.

Now we know that a longitudinal wave motion travels in the form of compressions and rarefactions which involve changes in the volume and density of the medium. As air possesses volume elasticity therefore sound comes to us from the source in the form of longitudinal waves only. As crests and troughs cannot be sustained in air, therefore sound cannot travel through the air in the form of transverse waves.

Sound waves are longitudinal mechanical waves that cannot travel in a vacuum. For example, two persons on the the surface of moon cannot talk to each other, as the moon has no atmosphere through which sound would travel **(Fig. 8.4)**.

■ SOME IMPORTANT TERMS CONNECTED WITH WAVE MOTION

- ❖ **Amplitude:** It is the maximum displacement that the particle of the medium in which the wave moves are displaced from their resting position as the wave train passes, it is equal to the half of the distance through with the particles vibrate.
- ❖ **Frequency:** The frequency of a particle is defined as the number of vibrations completed by a particle in one second or it is the number of waves (a pair of compression and rarefaction) crossing a point in one second. It is measured in cycles/second or Hertz and it is donated by (v).

CHAPTER 8: Sound Waves

- **Time period:** In wave motion, particles of medium execute simple harmonic motion or oscillatory motion, i.e., repeats its motion after a regular interval of time. This interval of time is called the time period. The time period of a wave is reciprocal to its frequency. In other words, it is the time taken by the wave to travel a distance equal to one wavelength. It is donated by 'T'. During one time period (T), the wave moves through a distance equal to one wavelength. Therefore the velocity (v) of wave.

$$\frac{V-\lambda}{T} = \lambda \upsilon$$

- **Wavelength:** Wavelength of a wave is equal to the length of one wave. It is defined as the distance between any two particles of the medium vibrating in the same phase. In the other wards, distance between two successive compressions or rarefaction is called the wavelength of the wave **(Fig. 8.5)**.
- **Velocity (V):** The velocity of waves varies with the medium through which the waves are passing and with the temperature of the medium. For Example, at 0°C, the velocity of sound waves in dry air is 1089 Ft/sec and at 200°C, it is 1126 Ft/sec.
  - In a rigid solid such as ivory, the sound travels at 3000 m/sec. In water at 190°C, the velocity of sound is 4794 Ft/sec.
  - The velocity of sound depends on the pressure and density of the medium through which it travels, i.e.,

$$V = \frac{P}{d}$$

here   P = Pressure, d = density
And   V = λ ν

If 'V' remains fixed, the wavelength will increase at increased temperature. Conversely, if the wavelength remains fixed, the frequency will increase with an increase in temperature.

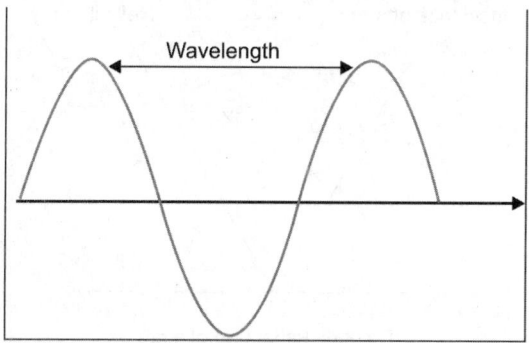

Fig. 8.5: Wavelength.

Out of three phases, solids metal conducts sound wave best and gases conducts sound waves poorly.

- **Intensity:** The intensity of sound depends on the amount of energy with which the sound waves strike the tympanic membrane of the intensitysity of sound is defined as the energy flow across a unit of area in a unit of time. In the MKS system, the unit of intensity of sound is watts per square meter.

The intensity of sound is inversely proportional to the square of the distance from the source, i.e.,

$$I \alpha 1/D^2$$

Where D is the distance from the source

Variations in the sound level are expressed in decibel (dB), i.e., intensity of sound with respect to various levels is expressed in dB.

The basic unit of sound intensity is 10^{-12} W/m^2 which is audible to the normal ear. Normal conversation is in the range below 60 dB and 70 dB, and heavy traffic produces a sound intensity of about 80 dB. At 120 dB a person feels discomfort whereas at 140 dB pain is experienced. A normal person can detect the sound of intensity between 10^{-12} W/m^2 and 1-12 W/m^2 (i.e., in the range of 0 to 120 dB).

■ WAVE PHENOMENON

Regardless of type, transverse or longitudinal, waves exhibit similar behavior. When any wave strikes a surface, the wave may be reflected, refracted, absorbed, transmitted, or diffracted or it may exhibit interference.

- **Reflection:** When waves or rays hit a flat surface they may be reflected back. For example; the echo exemplifies this phenomenon in sound waves **(Fig. 8.6)**.

In the case of perfect reflections, $\theta_1 = \theta_2$

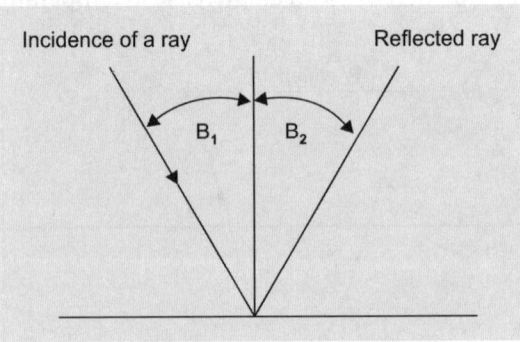

Fig. 8.6: Reflection of a ray.

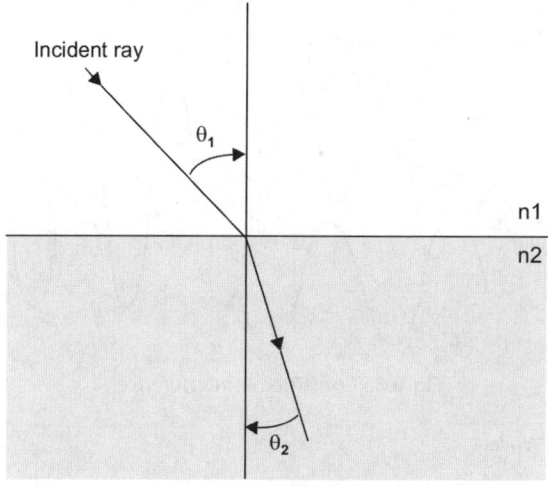

Fig. 8.7: Refraction of a ray.

- **Refraction:** When a wave or ray passes from one medium to another, its velocity may change, causing a change in the direction of the wave. The change in the direction is known as refraction (**Fig. 8.7**).
- **Absorption:** When a wave strikes a medium or a surface, some of the energy is absorbed and changed to heat. A piece of black cloth placed on snow on a bright sunny day may absorb sufficient radiant energy from the sun to melt the snow. For example, special materials used in the construction of soundproof rooms absorb rather than reflect the sound energy, transforming it into heat energy.
- **Transmission:** Waves or rays passing from a source of energy in a given medium move outward and are transmitted by the molecules of the medium. When the waves strike another medium, they are transmitted unchanged, if both media have the same refraction index.
- **Diffraction:** It is a term used to mean a departure from a straight line when waves meet and pass an obstacle or go through an aperture. In everyday speech, diffraction refers to the property of waves being able to "bend around corners".
- **Interference:** Interference may occur when more than one wave train is moving through the same medium. The effect can be demonstrated experimentally by propagating two wave trains in water that moves from opposite directions through an intervention. In the intersection area, the wave patterns are disrupted, but after

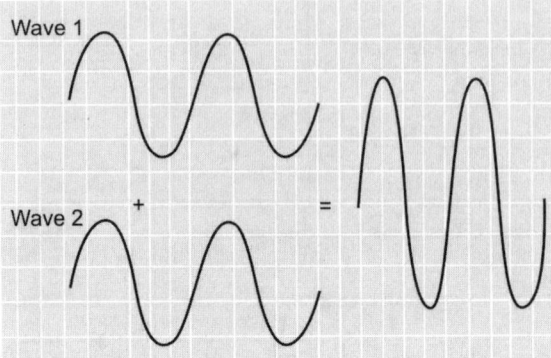

Fig. 8.8: Constructive interference.

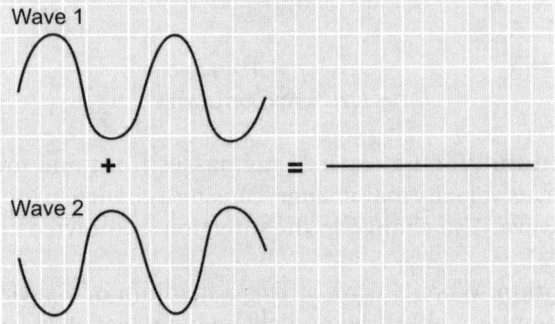

Fig. 8.9: Destructive interference.

passing the intersection the wavefront reappears in this original form.
- **Constructive:** When two small waves coming from opposite directions combine to form a large pulse and then reappear in their original form, it is called a constructive interference pattern **(Fig. 8.8)**.
- **Destructive:** When two transverse waves that are equal and opposite in direction meet, the upward and downward wave pulses cancel each other temporarily and a destructive interference pattern is formed **(Fig. 8.9)**.

■ CHARACTERISTICS OF SOUND

In our everyday life, we hear different types of sounds. Broadly, sound may be divided into two classes:
- ❖ **Musical sound:** Musical sound is a continuous and pleasing sound. It is produced by regular periodic vibrations. The sound produced by violin, guitar, piano, *ektara*, *tabla*, etc. is musical in nature.

CHAPTER 8: Sound Waves

❖ **Noise:** Every sound other than musical sound is noise. While the musical sound is pleasing, noise such as automobile horn is irritable and can adversely affect us. You may beware that the noise level in all metropolitan cities of or country has increased to alarming levels.

How do we differentiate among a variety of musical sounds such as from guitar, *sitar, veena*, tabla, etc? It can be done on the basis of three parameters, i.e., intensity, pitch, and quality (timber) as discussed below:

- **Intensity:** Intensity is defined as the energy carried by a wave in a unit of time across a unit area normal to the direction. It is measured in W/m^{-2}. Qualitatively, it is a measure of loudness. As we know,

$$I \alpha\ 1/r_2$$

For example, if 'r' increase, intensity decreases.

It is for this reason, that chirping of birds, the sound of the vehicle, or a cracker fad out **(Table 8.1)**.

- **Pitch:** The pitch of the sound is related to frequency. The greater the frequency of the sound waves the higher the pitch. If one inhales a quantity of helium and talks while exhaling it the voice sounds thin and piping. The velocity of sound in helium is greater than that in air and since the wavelength of the sounds produced by the vocal cords does not change, the frequency of the sound increases, and the pitch is raised.

- **Quality/Timber:** The quality of timber is the most important characteristic of a musical sound because it enables us to distinguish a sound produced by one musical instrument

Table 8.1: Intensities of sound waves generated from different sources.

Source	Intensity (wm^{-2})
Threshold of hearing	10^{-12}
Rusty waves	10^{-11}
Whisper, the intensity at eardrum	10^{-10}
Home	10^{-8}
Office	10^{-7}
Ordinary conversation	3.2×10^{-6}
Street traffic	10^{-15}
Busting cracker, at 1 m	8×10^{-5}
Jet take-off, at 7.8 m	105 W/m^2

from that of another instrument. The quality of a tone is dependent upon the frequencies that are integral multiples of the fundamental frequency. These frequencies are called harmonics. A "pure" tone depends upon the fundamental frequency only. The presence of different harmonics and their relative intensities introduce uniqueness in the sound produced by a particular source.

■ VOCALIZATION AND HEARING

Human beings have the ability to produce a variety of sounds. Physically this is possible because the vocal cords produce vibrations of various frequencies. Also air currents passing over the cords can produce a variety of intensities.

Vocalization

During normal breathing, the vocal cords are relaxed and air can pass easily through the larynx. A voiced sound is produced when the cords close off the larynx. As air is exhaled, pressure builds up behind the cords and escapes through them. This reduces the pressure on the back of the cords. When the pressure is reduced, the cords again close, the pressure again increases and the action is repeated. By the action of a series sound waves are produced, each with a specific frequency depending on the tension on the mass of the cord.

The character of the voice is influenced by the tension, thickness, and size of the cords as well as the size and shape of the throat, thorax, and paranasal sinuses. Thus in general, the frequency of sound is higher in women. This is because their vocal cords are lighter. Similarly, change of voice in adolescence is connected to the increase in mass that accompanies growth and development.

Hearing

Ear is responsible for hearing. The ear can be divided into three parts the external ear, the middle ear, and the inner ear The external ear is shaped like a cone, fixed at the periphery. At the end of the external ear lies the tympanic membrane, commonly called the eardrum. The middle ear contains the three ossicles the malleus, the incus, and the stapes. They stretch across the middle layer from the eardrum to the membrane of the head of the first ossicle. The hearing starts with the outer ear. When a sound is made outside the outer ear, the sound waves, or vibrations, travel down the external auditory canal and strike the eardrum (tympanic membrane). The eardrum vibrates. The vibrations are then passed to three tiny bones in the middle ear called the ossicles. The ossicles amplify the sound. Hearing results from stimulation of the nerve cells of the inner ear and the interpretation of these impulses in the brain.. The three ossicles are so mounted that the vibrations of the eardrum are transmitted to the last ossicles and at the oval window. This rocking motion, in turn, sets up pressure waves in the cochlear fluid in the inner ear. The cochlear of the inner ear is like a tapering coil.

This tube is divided into three canals which are filled with fluid. The partition between the two canals is madeup of the organ of Corti, which contains the sensory cells. Impulses from the nerve fibers, which are connected to sensory cells, project into the auditory center of the cerebrum.

Thus, the structure of the ear allows sound waves from the outside air to travel right up to the inner ear, where these vibrations are converted into nerve impulses. The external ear acts like a trumpet because of its conical shape and thus produces greater pressure on the eardrums. The middle ear exerts amplifying action, i.e., increases the intensity of the sound wave. The inner ear changes the vibrations in the fluid to specific increased impulses that are translated by the brain into the sound of varying pitch and loudness.

■ DOPPLER EFFECT

It was first described (1842) by Austrian physicist Christian Doppler. The apparent difference between the frequency at which sound or light waves leave a source and that at which they reach an observer, is caused by the relative motion of the observer and the wave source. You all must have heard the whistle of a moving train. What do you feel if the train approaches you? The pitch of the whistle seems to rise and when it goes away, the pitch appears to decrease. These apparent changes in the sound heard are caused due to Doppler effects.

In general, when the source approaches the listener or the listener approaches the source, or both approach each other, the apparent frequency is different than the actual frequency of the sound produced by the source. This change in frequency is known as the Doppler shift. Doppler shift can be used to measure the rate of blood flow. It is also used by obstetricians to detect fetal heartbeat or pulsation in the umbilical cord.

To detect the blood flow, a continuous ultrasound beam is sent to blood cells in an artery that is moving away from the source. The frequency of ultrasound received by the blood cells appears lower.

The apparent lowering of frequency is detected by the echoes sent by the blood cells, this helps estimate the rate of blood flow in an artery or any other organ of the human body and the heart rate of the fetus.

■ APPLICATIONS

Hearing Aids

Hearing aids are electronic devices consisting of a minute microphone that picks up sound waves and converts them into electric current. The current is amplified and passes to a miniature loudspeaker that fits into the ear.

Stethoscope

- ❖ The stethoscope is a familiar instrument for listening to sounds in the human body. This simple "hearing aid" permits a physician or nurse to listen to sounds made inside the body, primarily in the heart and lungs. This is called auscultation.
- ❖ The main parts of a modern stethoscope are the bell, which is either open or closed by a thin diaphragm, the tubing, and earpieces **(Fig. 8.10)**.
- ❖ A closed bell is an impedance matcher between the skin and the air and accumulates sound from the contact area. The skin under the open bell acts as a diaphragm. The skin diaphragm has a natural resonant frequency at which it most effectively transmits sounds.

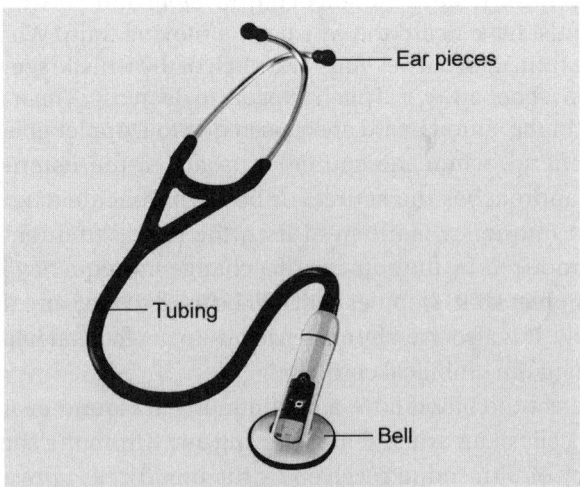

Fig. 8.10: Stethoscope.

It is used to hear the low-frequency heart murmurs.
- A crude open system used in midwifery is called a fetoscope and is used to hear the heart beats
- sounds of the baby in the pregnant uterus.
- In a stethoscope, we are dealing with a system that is closed at the far end by a pressure-sensitive diaphragm. It is desirable to have a bell with as small a volume as possible. The smaller the volume of gas, the greater the pressure changes for a given movement of the diaphragm at the end of the bell.
- The volume of tubes should also be small and there should be minimum frictional loss of sound due to the walls of tubes. Typically the length of the tube is 25 cm and its diameter is 0.3 cm.

Symbalophone

This instrument is made of two stethoscopes, one going to one ear, the other to the ear. Sounds coming from two regions may be heard at the same time and compared. An example of its use is the simultaneous comparison of the heart sounds of the fetus and mother.

Audiometry

- Audiometry is an apparatus for measuring the ability of the human ear to hear. Basically, measurements are made by determining the minimum intensity of sounds of various frequencies that are just distinguishable by the ear. The minimum intensity obtained is compared with that of the normal ear and is expressed in decibels.
- The audiometer is made to produce sounds of known frequency and intensity that are controlled by the operator. The patient is allowed to hear a sound at higher intensity, and then the intensity is gradually reduced to below the threshold for the patient. The intensity is then increased slowly until the patients just hear it. At that point, the patient signals the operator.
- Separate measurements are made for each ear and by the use of some special audiometers measurements of both air and bone conduction are made for each ear. The patient is tested throughout at intensities between 15 dB below the level which is the threshold for a normal ear and 95 dB above this level. The results of the measurements are recorded on a chart called an audiogram. Deviations from the zero point on these charts give a measure of hearing loss.
- Audiometers are of two types
  - Type 1 or Step Type: It has a limited number of specific discrete frequencies.
  - Type 2 or Sweep Type: It has a continuous range of frequencies.

- Frequencies frequently used in testing hearing are 125, 250, 500, 750, 1000, 2000, 3000, 4000, 6000, 8000 cps.

Speech Audiometry

❖ In order for a person to understand the spoken word he must be able to hear at least in the middle of the audiometer range, that is 500, 1000, and 2000 cps. The hearing level for these three frequencies is close to a person's hearing level for speech.

❖ The hearing level for speech can be measured by a test that uses tape-recordings of certain selected words of syllables, such as railroad, in which six such words are presented to the person being tested each time at a successively lower intensity level of 4 dB until the words are no longer heard by him.

❖ The intensity at which the person can repeat one-half of the words is accepted or is considered to be his speech reception threshold (SRT). The difference between this intensity level and the normal average SRT gives an indication of the person's hearing level of speech.

❖ By using a risk of phonetically balanced (PB) monosyllabic words, more information about a person's hearing may be obtained. The PB lists contain 50 words each and represent a frequency of sounds of speech that approximate those found in normal English conversation. A list of words is presented to the person at a uniform intensity. The percentage of words that the person can repeat correctly is called the discrimination score (DS). The average DS for loud sounds (85 dB), for normal sounds (70 dB), and for faint sounds (55 dB) is a practical measure of a person's ability to hear in everyday situations. The score is known as Davis Social Adequacy Index (SAI). The hearing ranges between 94 and 1000. The SAI score that represents the lower limit for social adequacy of the hearing is considered to be 33. A person within this range can understand that only amplified shouted speech may not be understood **(Table 8.2)**.

Table 8.2: Interpreting the hearing loss based on audiometry results.

Results	Interpretation
> 25 dB but not > 40 dB	Slight hearing loss
>40 dB but not > 55 dB	Mild hearing loss
>55 dB but not > 90 dB	Marked hearing loss
70 dB but not > 90 dB	Severe hearing loss

Applications

- Ear covers are recommended for employers who work in nosy locations.
- Airplane field attendants wear covers during landing and take-off of airplanes. Hearing protection is exposed for prolonged period to noises louder than 85 dB for frequencies above 150 cps.

Sonar Navigation and Ranging

During World War I, a technique called sound ranging was developed to locate the position of enemy guns by using a technique to detect the sound of cannon in action. This has led to the development of sonar (sound) navigation and ranging. In sonar, high-frequency sound waves are sent towards the target, and reflected sound is detected. The time taken by sound wave in this round trip gives an idea about the distance of the target **(Fig. 8.11)**.

$$V = \frac{x+x}{t}$$
$$v \times t = 2x$$
$$x = \frac{vt}{2}$$

Since velocity is known, distance can be calculated by measuring time.

Ultrasonic Sound Waves

Ultrasonic wave is defined as inaudible sound with high frequency for human, the frequency of which generally exceeds 20 kHz. Ultrasonic waves penetrate tissue and are scattered and absorbed within it. The scattered and reflected ultrasound contains information about the form and structure of the tissue. This ultrasound signal is converted into a visible image using specialized computer techniques, which is called ultrasound imaging.

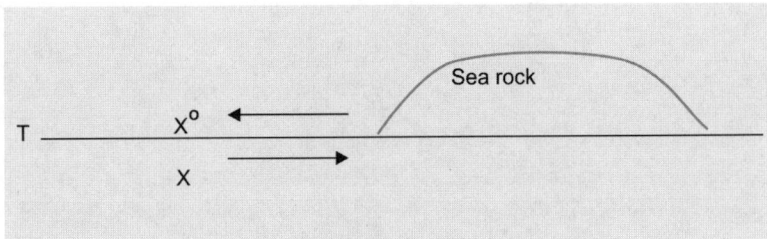

Fig. 8.11: Sonar navigation.

Production of ultrasonic sound waves: These waves are produced by:
- Magnetostrictive devices depend upon changes in the length of metals such as nickel when magnetized.
- Devices that utilize a crystal depend upon the crystal's exhibiting a piezoelectric reaction. This reaction is the movement of the crystal when a current is passed into it. The device, whether a moving crystal or metal, has a vibrating head known as the transducer, which produces the beam of ultrasonic sound waves.
  - **Adverse effects of the ultrasonic sound waves:** In brief, the effects of high-frequency ultrasonic sound are heating, paralytic and lethal effects.
  - **Heating:** Lipids and proteins have been shown to exhibit an increase in temperature when subjected to ultrasonic sound waves.
  - **Paralytic:** Paralysis of hind legs has been reported. Human beings exposed to ultrasonic fields for long periods of time may develop a loss of equilibrium and an inability to concentrate.
  - **Lethal:** Lethal effects have been reported in studies on large protozoa, red blood cells, and some bacteria.

Uses of Ultrasound

- **Ultrasound diathermy** is helpful in the treatment of joint disease and joint stiffness **(Fig. 8.12)**. Ultrasound waves interact with tissue primarily by microscopic motion of tissue particles. As these waves move through the tissue, the regions of compressions and rarefaction cause pressure differences in adjacent regions of the tissue.

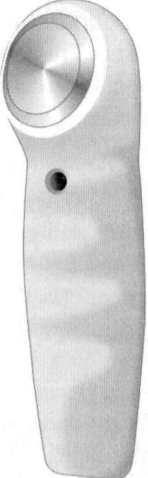

Fig. 8.12: Diathermy.

This results in stretching of stiff regions and gives relief to the patient. However, one has to be careful because if the stretching exceeds the elastic limit of the tissue, it may rupture. That is why the eardrum can be ruptured by a very intense sound.

- **Ultrasound:**
  - It mainly works upon the transmission and reflection properties of sound waves.
  - The other thing is change in velocity of sound waves in different mediums thus changing frequency, pitch, and direction.
  - Physics of ultrasound used in sonography: In general, pulses of ultrasound are transmitted into the body by placing the vibrating crystal in close contact with the skin, using water or a jelly paste to eliminate the air between the crystal and skin. This gives the good coupling at the skin and greatly increases the transmission of the ultrasound the pulse serves as a detector. The signals received are amplified and displayed on an oscilloscope. This procedure is called the A scanning method of ultrasound diagnosis. For many clinical purposes, A scans have been largely replaced by B scans. The B scan method is used to obtain two-dimensional views of the internal organs or the body. The principles of the B scan are the same as for the A scan except that the transducer is moved. A storage oscilloscope is used so that is lasting image can be formed and photography can be made.
  - **The main uses of ultrasound in healthcare practices are:**
    - Sonography is used to assess the fetal well-being during pregnancy as well as used to diagnose several medical illnesses like cirrhosis of the liver, tumors of organs in the abdominal or pelvic cavity, obstruction of intestine, etc.
    - **Echocardiography:** A technique that transmits ultrasonic signals into the tissues and utilized a receiver that record changes in blood velocity have been employed to diagnose heart conditions.
    - Use in diagnosing eye diseases like cataract, measuring the thickness of cornea, the thickness of vitreous humor, etc.
    - **Fetal heart monitoring:** Fetal heart monitor has the ability to reflect ultrasonic sound signals so that the fetal heart beat in as early a period as the 12th week of pregnancy can be detected.
    - **Echoencephalography:** This technique is based on partial reflection of sound at the interface of two media. It is used to detect brain tumors. In this process, the ultrasound pulses are sent in the skull slightly above the ear, and echoes from

the left side of the head are compared with those from the right side.

■ NOISE POLLUTION AND ITS PREVENTION

Noise is often defined as 'unwanted sound' but this definition is subjective to the fact that one man's sound may be another man's noise. Perhaps a better definition of noise is "wrong sound in the wrong place, at the wrong time." Man is living in an increasingly noisy environment. Noise pollution is displeasing human, animal or machine-created sound that disrupts the activity or balance of human or animal life. The word noise comes from the Latin word nausea meaning seasickness.

Sources of Noise

The source of most outdoor noise worldwide is transportation systems, including motor vehicle noise, aircraft noise, and rail noise. Poor urban planning may give rise to noise pollution since side-by-side industrial and residential buildings can result in noise pollution in the residential area.

Other sources of indoor and outdoor noise pollution are car alarms, emergency service sirens, office equipment, factory machinery, construction work, groundskeeping equipment, barking dogs, appliances, power tools, lighting hum, audio entertainment systems, loudspeakers, and noisy people.

Human Health Effects of Noise

Noise health effects are both health and behavioral in nature. The unwanted sound is called noise. This unwanted sound can damage physiological and psychological health. Noise pollution can cause annoyance and aggression, hypertension, high-stress levels, tinnitus, hearing loss, sleep disturbances, and other harmful effects. Furthermore, stress and hypertension are the leading causes of health problems, whereas tinnitus can lead to forgetfulness, severe depression, and at times panic attacks.

Chronic exposure to noise may cause noise-induced hearing loss. Older males exposed to significant occupational noise demonstrate significantly reduced hearing sensitivity than their non-exposed peers, though differences in hearing sensitivity decrease with time and the two groups are indistinguishable by age 79. A comparison of Maaban Tribesmen, who were insignificantly exposed to transportation or industrial noise, to a typical US population showed that chronic exposure to moderately high levels of environmental noise contributes to hearing loss.

High noise levels can contribute to cardiovascular effects and exposure to moderately high levels during a single eight hour period causes a statistical rise in blood pressure of five to ten points and an increase in stress and vasoconstriction leading to the increased blood pressure noted above as well as to the increased incidence of coronary artery disease. Noise pollution is also a cause of annoyance. A 2005 study by Spanish researchers found that in urban areas households are willing to pay approximately four Euros per decibel per year for noise reduction.

Hearing Loss

Hearing loss is inability to partially or completely hear sound in one or both of ears. Hearing loss typically occurs gradually over time. It can be Mild (26-40 decibel), Moderate (41-55 decibel), and Severe (more than 71 decibels) hearing loss.

A person's auditory system consists of the outer ear, middle ear, inner ear and acoustic nerve. The sound wave comes to outer ear then hit on eardrum causing vibration to the drum. This vibration moves to inner ear through bones of middle ear. Where it is converted in nerve impulse by organ of Corti. From there these impulses carried to brain via acoustic nerve. When one of these parts is not working in an optimal way, a hearing loss can occur. While hearing loss can range from mild to profound, there are four classifications that all hearing losses fall under.

There are four types of hearing loss sensorineural, conductive, mixed (sensorineural and conductive) and auditory neuropathy spectrum disorder.

Sensorineural Hearing Loss

Sensorineural hearing loss happens when there's damage to inner ear (cochlea) structures or in the acoustic nerve pathways to the brain. Damage to these structures can occur due to exposure to loud noises, illness (meningitis), ototoxic medications, or it can happen simply due to genetics or the aging process(Presbycusis).

Sensorineural hearing loss is permanent, and treatments include the use of hearing aids and cochlear implants.

Conductive Hearing Loss

A conductive hearing loss occurs when something prevents sound from passing through the outer or middle ear and into the inner ear.

This can occur when earwax or fluid builds up in the ear canal, or when there is damage to the eardrum or bones in the middle ear. There may also be a birth defect that prevents sound waves from entering the ear to stimulate the acoustic nerve, such as atresia or microtia.

Treatments may include surgery to repair structural abnormalities, a procedure to remove blockages, or the use of a hearing aid, cochlear implant. A cochlear implant is a small electrical machine placed under the skin behind the ear. It translates sound vibrations into electrical signals that brain can interpret as meaningful sound.

When this type of hearing loss occurs, patient may find it difficult to hear soft or muffled sounds. So nurse should use clear and higher pitched sound.

Mixed Hearing Loss

In some cases, a person may be suffering from both a sensorineural and conductive hearing loss. Mixed hearing loss affects both the inner ear and outer or middle ear, and as such, it can lead to a more profound hearing loss.

Treatments will vary depending on the severity of the hearing loss, but in addition to a surgical procedure, hearing aids and cochlear implants may be necessary.

Auditory Neuropathy Spectrum Disorder

Sometimes sound is able to enter an ear normally and reach the acoustic nerve, but there is a problem when the sound is transmitted to the brain. This hearing loss is known as auditory neuropathy spectrum disorder (ANSD).

ANSD can occur due to various reasons. In some cases, the hair cells of the inner ear are damaged and are unable to properly transmit sound information to the brain. Sometimes a genetic mutation is the cause of this hearing loss, and other times damage to the auditory nerve can lead to ANSD.

People with ANSD may seem to have normal hearing sensitivity on a hearing test, but they may struggle to understand spoken words. In some cases, a hearing aid or cochlear implant paired with a hearing assistive technology (HAT) system can help mitigate the negative effects of this hearing loss. However, more severe cases, in which the person has great difficulty understanding speech, may require the use of a visual communication technique, like sign language or a picture exchange communication system (PECS).

Physical exam

A physical exam can help differentiate SNHL from conductive hearing loss. A doctor will search for inflammation, fluid or earwax build-up, damage to your eardrum, and foreign bodies.

Tuning forks

A tuning fork test as an initial screening. In Weber's test a 512 Hz tuning fork stroked softly and places it near the midline of forehead. If the sound is louder in affected ear, hearing loss is likely conductive. If sound is louder in unaffected ear, hearing loss is likely sensorineural. Whereas in Rinne test a tuning fork stroked and places it against mastoid bone behind ear until person no longer hear the sound. Then the tuning fork is moved in front of ear canal until person can't hear the sound. If anyone has SNHL, will be able to hear the tuning fork better in front of your ear canal than against your bone.

Audiogram

During the test, headphones are worn in a soundproof booth. Tones and words will be played into each ear at different volumes and frequencies. The test helps find the quietest sound that anyone can hear and specific frequencies of hearing loss as mentioned earlier.

Precautions

- ❖ Use safety equipment if you work in areas with loud noises, and wear earplugs when you swim and go to concerts.
- ❖ Keep your headphone volume under 60 percent.
- ❖ Consult a doctor before starting a new medication.
- ❖ Have regular hearing tests if you work around loud noises, swim often, or go to concerts on a regular basis.
- ❖ Avoid prolonged exposure to loud noises and music.
- ❖ Seek help for ear infections. They may cause permanent damage to the ear if they are left untreated.

Prevention of Noise Pollution

A variety of approaches may be needed to prevent and control the noise pollution; there are as follows:
- ❖ **Carefully planning of cities:** In planning the cities, the following measures should be taken to reduce noise:
  - Division of the cities into zones with separation of areas concerned with industry and transportation.
  - The separation of the residential area from the main street by means of wide green belts. Houses front should lie not less than 15 meters from the road and the intervening space should be thickly planted with trees and bushes.

- Widening of the main street to reduce the penetration of noise into the dwelling area.
- **Control of the vehicles:** Heavy vehicles should not be routed into narrow streets. Vehicular traffic on residential streets should be reduced. The indiscriminate blowing of the horn and use of pressure horn should be prohibited.
- **To improve acoustic insulation of building:** From the acoustic standpoint, the best arrangement is the construction of detached buildings rather than a single large building or one that is continuous. Installation that produces noise or disturb the occupant within the dwelling should be prohibited. Buildings should be soundproof where necessary.
- **Industries and railways:** Control of the noise at the source is possible in industries. The special area must be earmarked, outside residential areas, for industries, railways, marshaling yards, and smaller installations. When these demands cannot be met, a protective green belt must be laid down between the installations and residential areas.
- **Protection of exposed persons:** Hearing protection is recommended for all workers who are consistently exposed to noise louder than 85 decibels in the frequency band above 150 Hz. Workers must be regularly rotated from noisy areas to comparatively quiet posts in factories. Periodical audiogram check-ups and use of earplugs must be ensured. Muffs are also essential as the situation demands.
- **Legislation:** Many adapted legislation provided for controls that are applicable to a wide variety of sources. Workers have the right to claim compensation if they have suffered a loss of ability to understand speech.
- **Education:** No noise abatement program can be successful without people's participation. Therefore, their education through all available media is needed to highlight the importance of noise as a community hazard.

■ QUESTIONS

Q.1: Use of stethoscope for listening to sounds for human body.

Q.2: During pregnancy ultrasound examination is advised instead of an X-ray examination.

Q.3: Discuss about the hearing aid and transmission of sound in the ear.

■ BIBLIOGRAPHY

1. Berglund B, Lindvall T, Schwela D, et al. "World Health Organization: Guidelines for Community Noise". World Health Organization, 1999.
2. Field JM. "Effect of personal and situational variables upon noise annoyance in residential areas". Journal of the Acoustical Society of America, 1993;93(5):2753-63.
3. Kryter, Karl D. The handbook of hearing and the effects of noise: physiology, psychology, and public health. Boston: Academic Press,1994.
4. National Research Council (US) Committee on Disability Determination for Individuals with Hearing Impairments; Dobie RA, Van Hemel S, editors. Hearing Loss: Determining Eligibility for Social Security Benefits. Washington (DC): National Academies Press (US); 2004. 2, Basics of Sound, the Ear, and Hearing. Available from: https://www.ncbi.nlm.nih.gov/books/NBK207834/
5. Park K. Park's Textbook of Preventive and Social Medicine. 20th edition. Jabalpur: Banarsidas Bhanot Publishers, 2009.
6. Passchier-VW, Passchier WF. "Noise exposure and public health". Environ Health Perspect. 2000;108(1):123-31.
7. Paul Davidovits, Waves and Sound, Editor(s): Paul Davidovits, Physics in Biology and Medicine (Fifth Edition), Academic Press, 2019,Pages 173-92. https://doi.org/10.1016/B978-0-12-813716-1.00012-4.
8. Walker JR, Fahy F. Fundamentals of noise and vibration. London: E & FN Spon, 1998.

CHAPTER 9

Electricity and Electromagnetism

Suresh K Sharma, Navjot Kaur

CHAPTER OUTLINE

- Types of Electricity
- Sources of Electric Current
- Effects of Electric Current
- Effects of Electricity on the Human Body
- Magnetism
- Applications of the Magnet and Magnetism
- Electroencephalography (EEG)
- Electrocardiography (ECG)
- Phonocardiography
- Electromyography (EMG)
- Electromyography Pattern
- Electrostimulation
- Electroconvulsive Therapy (ECT)
- Electronic Cardiac Pacemaker
- Brain Pacemaker
- Defibrillation
- Automated External Defibrillator
- Magnetic Resonance Imaging (MRI)
- CAT Scan

■ INTRODUCTION

The phenomenon of electricity was known to the ancient Greeks, who observed in 600 BC, that a piece of amber, when rubbed vigorously with a woolen cloth would attract light particles of matter towards it. Gilbert is credited with gaining the term 'electric'. He called these substances that exhibited attraction forces for one another when rubbed, as 'electrics' from the Greek word for amber 'electron'.

A charge is an inherent property of matter. Just as the mass is responsible for the gravitational forces, charge is responsible for electric forces. The three most common particles are electrons, protons, and neutrons. Electrons are negatively charged and protons are positively charged while neutrons are neutral. Charge on an electron repels charge on another electron while it attracts a proton, i.e., similar charges repel each other while opposite charges attract. We can experience by rubbing two solid bodies against each other. If we pass a comb through dry hair, it becomes electrically charged and can attract pieces of paper. A sheet of paper becomes charged when it is passed through a printing machine.

■ TYPES OF ELECTRICITY

Basically, electricity is classified into two broad categories, i.e. electrostatics or static electricity and electrodynamics.
1. **Electrostatics or Static Electricity:** It is characterized by the accumulation of charges of electricity on the surface of substances.
2. **Electrodynamics:** It is characterized by the flow of electrons through a conductor.

Electrostatics (Static Electricity)
- If a glass is rubbed with a silk cloth and suspended, it will be repelled by a rod similarly treated when the second rod is brought close to the first.
- A hard-rubber rod rubbed with wool is similarly repelled by another hard rubber rod.
- If the glass rod is placed near the suspended rubber rod, however, the two are attracted. These are examples of the production of electricity by friction **(Fig. 9.1)**.

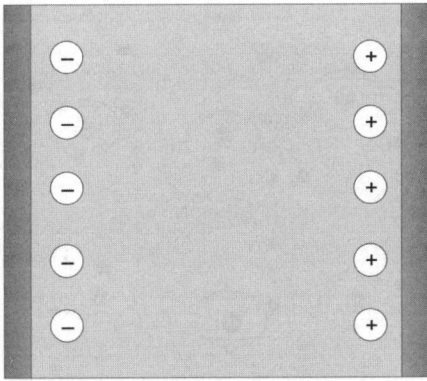

Charges build in static electricity

Fig. 9.1: Static electricity.

- For example, many of us have at one time or another experienced the shock of static electricity by walking across a thick rug and then touching a metal object such as a door knob or key in a lock.

Theory of Electrification

Static electricity is with respect to the structure of the atom. All atoms are made of a closely packed nuclei having a positive charge and containing neutrons and protons. Around the nucleus are electrons with negative charges.

The electrons are found at various energy levels or in orbits at a distance from the nucleus. In an object such as a copper wire, which is made-up of many copper atoms, it is conceivable that electrons in the outer regions of the atoms might move at random from one atom to another, if an electron leaves the outer region of one atom, another electron must move in from a different atom to maintain the neutrality of first atom **(Fig. 9.2)**. These are called free electrons.

It is generally assumed that non-electrified or uncharged objects possess equal numbers of positive and negative charges. When friction is applied, in the case of the glass rod rubbed with silk, some negative charges (electrons) are apparently transferred from the glass to the silk. This leaves the glass rod with a net positive charge and the silk with an equal net negative charge. Similarly, the hard rubber rod receives negative charges from the wool and leaves the wool positively charged. It is theorized that free electrons are actually transferred in the rubbing process. If a substance receives extra free

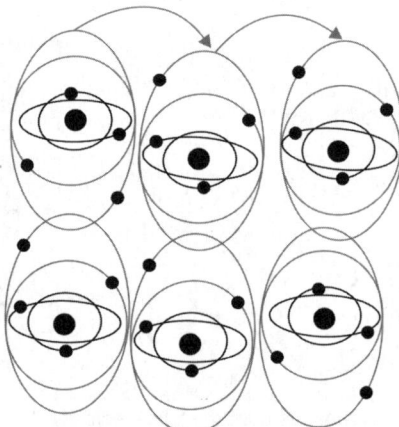

Fig. 9.2: Theory of electrification.

electrons from another, the substance is said to be negatively charged. If an object loses free electrons, it is said to be positively charged.

Coulomb's Law

It states that "force of attraction or repulsion between the two charges is directly proportional to the product of the charges and inversely proportional to the square of the distance between them".

$$F = \frac{KQ_1Q_2}{r_2}$$

Mathematically, here Q_1 and Q_2 are the charges on the particles, 'r' is the distance between them, and 'K' is the constant of proportionality which depends upon the medium.

Conduction

A piece of matter of any size contains billions of atoms, and each atom contains a positively charged nucleus and several electrons around it. In gases, the atoms almost do not interact with each other or a negligible interaction is there. In solids and liquids, the interaction is stronger. In some of them, the outer electrons of each atom are weakly bound to it (called free electrons) and have a high conductivity, called conductors. In another type of material, all electrons are tightly bound to their respective atoms or molecules, i.e. there are no free electrons, called insulators. There is one more type of material, that behave like insulators at 0K, but at higher temperatures, few electrons are able to free themselves from atoms and thus conduct electricity, called semiconductors.

We can summarize, that substances that transmit electrons freely are good conductors of electricity. Examples of such good conductors are metals and aqueous solutions of acids, bases, and salts. Out of the metals, silver is the best conductor, however, because of the cost factor, copper is mostly used **(Fig. 9.3)**.

Substances that do not transmit electrons freely are called insulators. A few examples are dry air, rubber, and glass. Dry wood, distilled water and alcohol are intermediate in action and are called poor conductors.

Semiconductors, the substances, those are intermediate with respect to conducting electrons. Very common examples are germanium and silicon mainly used in transistors **(Fig. 9.4)**.

Examples

- ❖ Because the water for household use almost always contains some salts in solution. It conducts electricity.

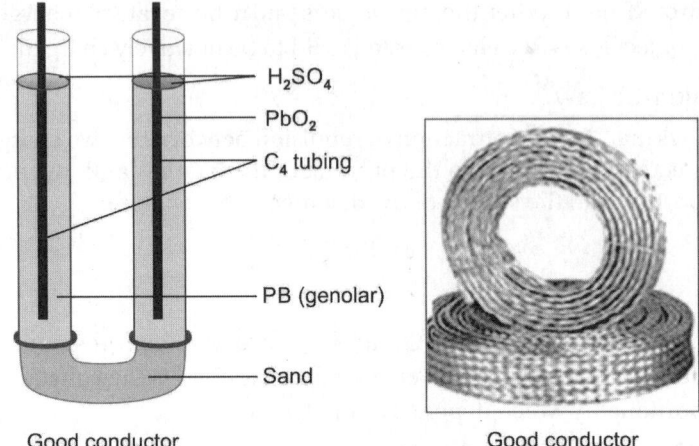

Good conductor   Good conductor

Fig. 9.3: Good conductors.

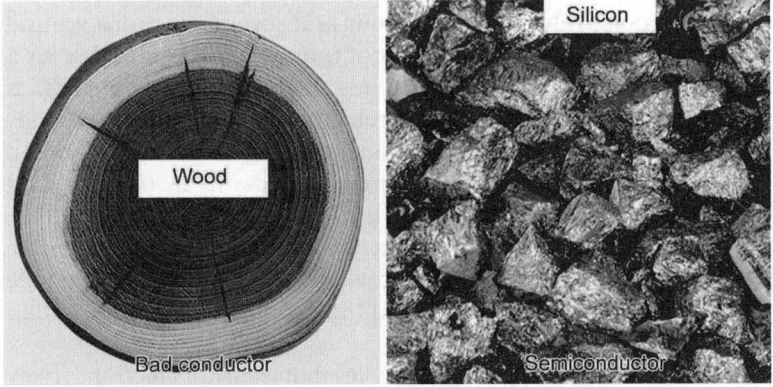

Fig. 9.4: Bad and semiconductor.

- A frayed, wet electric cord in which the wires are exposed may shock a person touching it.
- Electrocution has occurred from touching a faulty switch or the chain of an electric fixture with wet hands.
- Since the tissues of the human body are bathed by a saline solution, the body itself is capable of conducting electricity. This is the basis for many treatments and diagnostic tests.

Induction

It is also possible to electrify objects by a process known as induction.

- **Process of induction:** In this process, if a negatively charged rod is brought close to an uncharged insulated conductor, the electrons on the side of the conductor nearer the rod are repelled, and move toward the other side of the conductor, leaving the side nearer the rod positively charged. Actually, there is no gain or loss of electrons, but rather a separation of two kinds of charges. If the conductor is then grounded (connected to earth by a wire) or touched with the finger, the electrons pass to ground. In this way the conductor retains the positive charges. For example, lightning rod.

❖ In the atmosphere, positive charges accumulate on moving "thunder clouds". Under the cloud on the surface of the earth, a corresponding negative charge is induced. As the cloud begins to move toward the earth, the tension between its charges and those on the earth's surface increases. The air becomes ionized, it is no longer a good insulator, and the charges unite with a flash of light and a release of heat energy that is commonly called lightening. A lightning rod is an example of a pointed conductor that extends from damp or wet ground to the air above buildings. The lightning rod causes some of the charge induced in the earth by the charges on the cloud to pass into the air, thus reducing the potential difference between the cloud and earth to a level at which no lightning is produced **(Fig. 9.5)**.

Discharging of Charged Bodies

There are three ways in which a charged object may discharge its electricity. These are by spark, by brush discharge, and by conduction. The spark is disruptive and causes a breakdown of the surrounding medium with the emission of radiant energy. It occurs from highly polished spherical knobs that have dry air between them **(Fig. 9.6)**.

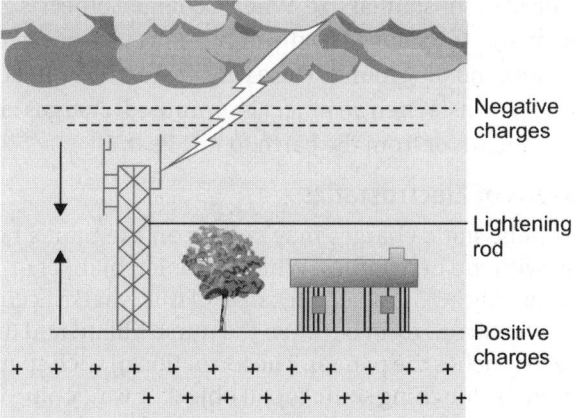

Fig. 9.5: Lightening rod.

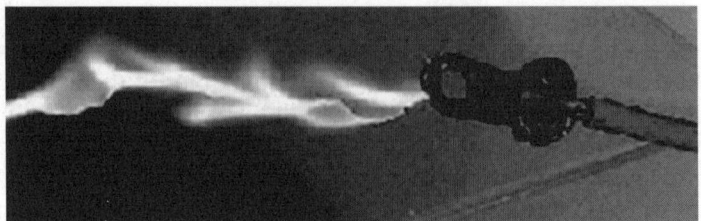

Fig. 9.6: Discharge by spark.

In a brush discharge, on the other hand, charges accumulate unevenly and are concentrated at projections and sharp points. The air molecules next to these "brush points" become charged with the same charge as is on the points. The air is then repelled from the point since both charges are the same and this actually creates a breeze, moving the air back from the point of discharge.

Electrostatic precipitation: It is used in industry to reduce air pollution and to recover material that would otherwise be lost in smoke. In this procedure, metallic points or small wires that are highly charged by induction from an electrostatic machine are placed in smoke stacks. When the wires are charged, the air in the chimney is repelled and the particles in the smoke is "precipitated out". Lightning rods also act by brush discharge during a storm when no lightning occurs. Discharges may be made also by conduction through a process called grounding. In this procedure, the discharge is practically instantaneous. Grounding is the process of removing the excess charge on an object by means of the transfer of electrons between it and another object of substantial size. When a charged object is grounded, the excess charge is balanced by the transfer of electrons between the charged object and the ground. The earth is said to be a great reservoir for excess electrons. When an object is grounded, charges either pass from it to the earth or from the earth to it **(Fig. 9.7)**.

Applications of Electrostatics

❖ In hospitals, static charges may collect on the hands because of friction with the bedclothes. When a woolen blanket or a sheet is rubbed briskly across a bed. Because of this, sparks accompanied by mild shock may form between the nurse's hand and the patient when she touches the patient. The formation of such sparks can be prevented by touching some metal object or water pipe with a flat hand. In this way, excess electrons are conducted to the ground.

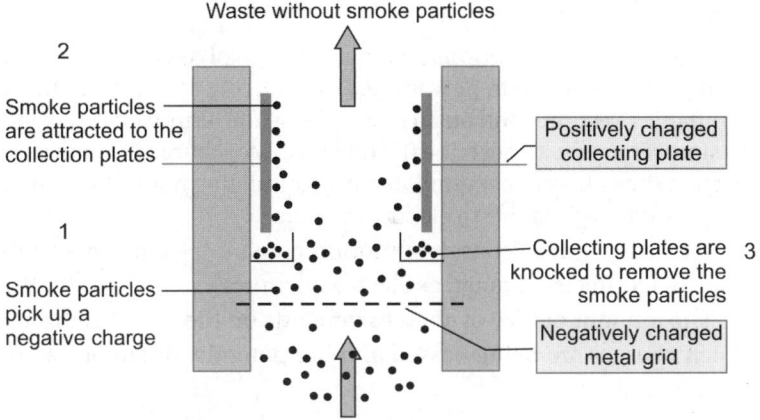

Fig. 9.7: Electrostatic precipitation.

- The use of woolen blankets on beds of patients in an oxygen tent and in operating rooms is sometimes forbidden for the same reason. Tests indicate that potential differences between the floor and the operating room table of as much as 10,000 volts may be produced in moving a woolen blanket when it is rubbed briskly over a rubber-covered mattress. The formation of sparks would be extremely dangerous in an atmosphere filled with explosive mixtures of anesthetic such as ether and air.
- The use of silk, nylon, or Dacron uniforms in the operating rooms is forbidden in some hospitals.
- Rubber-soled shoes are not recommended since they insulate the wearer from the floor and cause charges to accumulate on the person.
- Because dry air tends to promote an accumulation of static electricity, high relative humidity in the operating room will help to prevent spark formation.
- It is the practice in some operating rooms to wrap a damp cloth around the feet of the operating room tables to allow for easier passage of the charges from the table to the floor.
- All electrical equipment used in the operating room, including the operating table, should be grounded. Grounding is produced by means of a chain or cable leading from the apparatus to a water pipe or radiator that makes contact with the earth.
- Articles should be checked periodically with conductivity tests which can detect how well one object can conduct away static electric charges that tend to accumulate on its surface.

Electrodynamics

Most practical applications of electricity involve electric current, from your table lamp to power lines transferring energy from power companies to homes and businesses. We use the term 'electric current' or 'simply current' to describe the rate of flow of charge through some space. When charges accumulate on a conducting body, they tend to move and this gives rise to electric current.

We can say that "charge in motion constitutes current and the study of its effects is known as electrodynamics".

The amount of flow of charges depends on the material through which charges are being passed and the potential difference across the material.

Current

Consider two points between which a potential difference exists and suppose they are connected by a copper wire. Free electrons tend to flow from a lower potential point to a higher potential point (opposite to the direction of the electric field). Current is assumed to be opposite to the direction of flow of negative charges and in direction of flow of positive charges **(Fig. 9.8)**.

"The rate of flow of charge in a conductor is known as current". Mathematically, we can write current

$$I = \frac{Q}{t}$$

Where

I = current
Q = change
t = time

We can visualize the electric current as the number of electrons that pass through any section per second. The practical unit of current is ampere, which is donated by 'A'.

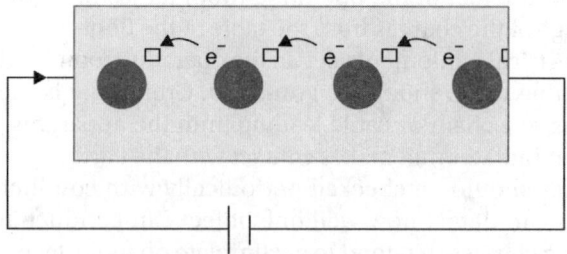

Fig. 9.8: Flow of charges.

Battery and Electromotive Force

Electromotive force is defined as the electric potential produced by either electrochemical cell or by changing the magnetic field. Electromotive force is the commonly used acronym for electromotive force. A battery is an electrochemical device that maintains a potential difference between its two terminals. The battery's internal mechanism exerts forces on charges of battery material so that positive charges move towards the positive terminal of the battery and negative charges towards the negative terminal of the battery. And thus, creates a potential difference between its two terminals.

Electromotive force is defined as the work done on a unit charge. The free electrons in conductors are the charges constituting electric current in a circuit. In addition to these free electrons, some sort of force is needed to push the electrons along the circuit. This force comes from the potential difference or electromotive force. It is measured in volt.

Resistance

Just as friction opposes the mechanical motion, the opposition to the flow of electric current in an electric circuit is known as resistance **(Fig. 9.9)**.

The practical unit of electrical resistance is the ohm. One ohm is that resistance across which a potential difference of 1 volt produces a current of 1 ampere. The resistance of a conductor wire depends on its length, area of cross-section, the nature of the material, and temperature.

To understand EMF and resistance, we can form an analogy between water pipes and electric wires. Just as higher the height of the water tank or more pressure in the pipe, water will flow with more speed; higher potential difference leads to higher current.

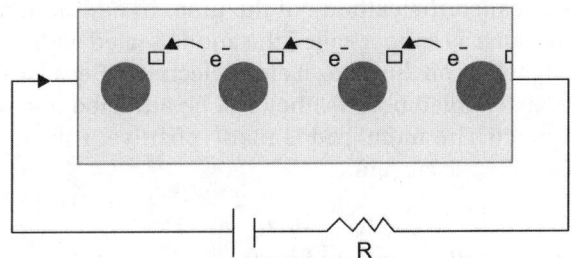

Fig. 9.9: Electronic circuit with resistance.

Suppose if we insert a few pieces of cotton in a pipe, water will flow with a comparatively slower speed now; similarly, the resistance is, depends on the material and opposes the flow of charges.

Ohm's Law

The relationship between resistance, voltage, and current was formulated by Ohm. It is stated as follows:

"The current in a conductor is linearly proportional to the difference of potential between any two points and inversely proportional to the resistance, provided physical conditions such as temperature, pressure, area of cross-section, etc. remain unchanged".

Mathematically, we can write:

$$I = \frac{V}{R}$$

Here 'I' is current in amperes, 'V' is voltage in volts, 'R' is resistance in ohms.

■ SOURCES OF ELECTRIC CURRENT

Since an electric current exists only when electrons move through a conductor. A continuous source of energy must be available to keep the electrons in motion. This energy may be of various types such as radiant, thermal, chemical, mechanical, or magnetic.

Radiant source of electricity: When light rays fall upon a clean metallic surface such as a film of potassium or sodium, electrons are emitted by the surface of the metal. This phenomenon is called the photoelectric effect. In addition to potassium and sodium, lithium, cesium, and selenium have photo-emissive properties. They emit electrons when light falls on their surfaces.

Device: These electrons can be made to form an electric current through a device called a photoelectric cell **(Fig. 9.10)**. The cell consists of a tube containing a curved plate of photosensitive metal. This plate is called the cathode of the tube. In addition, there is a rod of metal such as copper called the anode sealed within the tube. When the light falls on the plate, it emits electrons. Because electrons are negatively charged objects, they will be attracted to a positively charged object. The metal rod is made positive. Essentially, this produces an electric current.

Uses

- ❖ Automatic illumination of buildings
- ❖ Traffic signals
- ❖ Automatic opening and closing of doors as persons approach them.

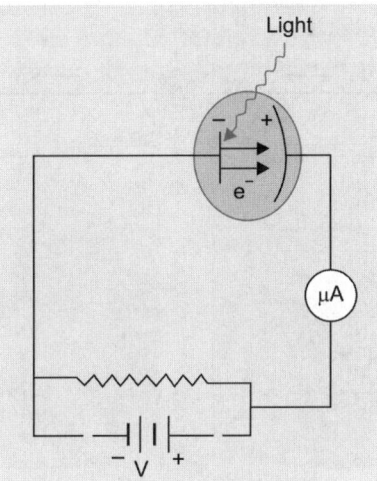

Fig. 9.10: Photoelectric cell.

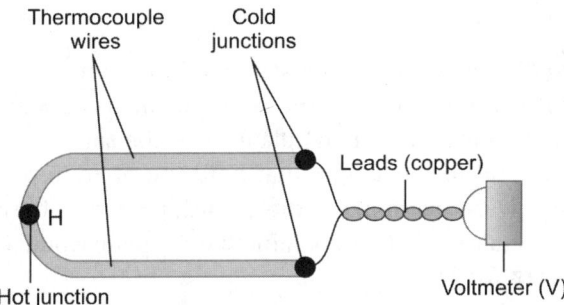

Fig. 9.11: Thermocouple.

Thermal source of electricity: Heat can also be used to develop small amounts of electricity. If a wire loop consisting of a piece of copper joined to a piece of iron is heated at one junction, a current will flow through the loop. Such a loop of dissimilar metals joined at both ends is called a thermocouple **(Fig. 9.11)**.

The flow of electrons continues as long as one junction is at a higher temperature than the other. The thermocouple is used to measure high temperatures. It is sometimes used to control the supply of fuel to a gas furnace. It cannot be used for producing large amounts of electricity continuously. It may be used to detect heat from a distant object. The degree of heat is ascertained by measuring the amount of current produced.

Chemical source of electric current: Certain metals placed in a solution of acids, bases, or salts (electrolytes) give off electrons.

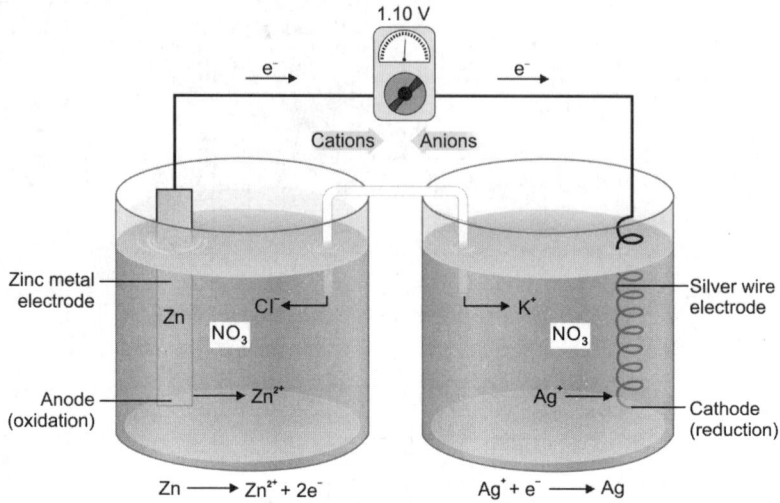

Fig. 9.12: Voltaic cell.

When two dissimilar metals are separated from one another by an electrolyte, a current will flow, for example, the orthopedic surgeon immobilizing bones with metal plates uses the same type of metal in the plate and in the screws that hold the plate in place. If the precautions were overlooked, the resulting current between two dissimilar metals might be so painful that the plate would have to be removed **(Fig. 9.12)**.

Voltaic cell: $Zn^{(-)}$ and $Cu^{(+)}$ in H_2SO_4

Magnetic and mechanical sources of electricity: Light, heat, and chemical energy can generate electricity, but the amounts are limited. To produce almost unlimited amounts of electricity, a method of making it by utilizing magnetism, specialty a magnetic field, is generally employed. The process can be traced back to two sides. In 1820, Oersted discovered the presence of a magnetic field around a wire coil carrying an electric current, and in 1931, Faraday discovered the flow of electric current when he moved a bar magnet through a wire coil. Faraday also found a flow of electricity as he withdrew the magnet. The motion of the electricity in the coil continued only while the magnet was in a motion and passed into or out of the coil. Thus, it was a comparatively simple method of producing electricity. Examples, generators or dynamo **(Fig. 9.13)**.

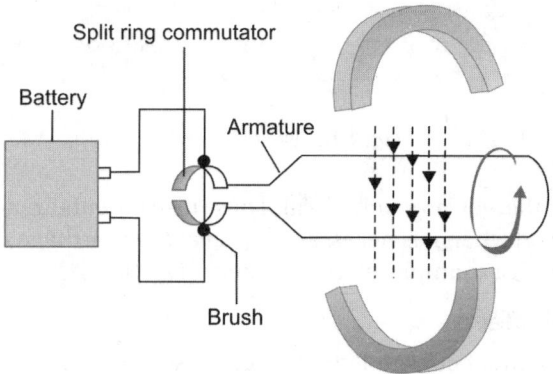

Fig. 9.13: Working of generators.

■ EFFECTS OF ELECTRIC CURRENT

As other forms of energy can be transformed into electrical energy, vice versa is also true. When an electric current passes through a conductor, a variety of effects may be produced. These effects may be described as radiant, thermal, chemical, mechanical, or magnetic.

Radiant Effects

- It is the transformation of electric energy into light energy.
- When the electrons in a circuit pass through a tungsten filament of an incandescent lamp, they heat the wire and give off electromagnetic waves of visible light.
- The incandescent filament in a 100-watt lamp produces a temperature of about 4,600 degrees Fahrenheit.
- If the filament were surrounded by air, the metal filament would oxidize and burn up at the temperature produced. For this reason, the air is removed from the bulb and an inert gas that does not support combustion is captured in the light bulb.
- Another example is fluorescent tubes.

Thermal Effects

- The flow of electrons through a conductor such as a special resistance wire produces heat.
- Electric hot plates, irons, toasters, heaters, heating pads, and electric cauterizes operate on this principle.
- Specially made surgical instruments operating on low amperage and high-frequency alternating currents may be used to coagulate tissues and small bleeding vessels during an operation. The current is discharged from the edges of the instrument directly to the

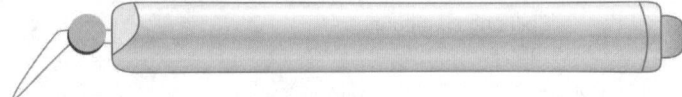

Fig. 9.14: Electric cautery.

tissues, thereby producing heat. These instruments are sometimes employed when it is necessary to prevent hemorrhage as in brain surgery. For example, electric cautery **(Fig. 9.14)**.

Chemical Effects

- When a direct current flows through a solution of an electrolyte, chemical changes occur.
- Electrolysis may be used to destroy the follicles of unwanted hair by causing the cells of the follicle to disintegrate chemically. Considerable skill is required to destroy the hair follicle by electrolysis without damaging the skin.
- Under certain conditions, the electric current is found in the circuits of private homes. An institution may be sufficient to cause death. When a person is standing in water, as may happen in a tub or shower, current travels rapidly from the appliance through the person towards the ground. This sudden passage of electricity may overstimulate the vagus nerve to the point of stopping the heart and death may result. Death may also occur from the chemical disintegration of the tissues through which the current passes.

Mechanical Effects

A generator is an apparatus for producing an induced current by rotating a wire loop through magnetic lines of force. A motor might be called a generator in reverse. The electric motor uses electrical energy produced by the generation to produce motion. Electric motors are used in an almost endless list of modern devices such as fans, refrigerators, sewing machines, sanders, polishers, and typewriters, and in the hospital for operating suction machines, centrifuges, and many other therapeutic apparatus. Basically, the motor consists of a rotating coil in a magnetic field. A current is passed through the wire coil of the motion, and this coil, known as the armature, rotates to produce power that can be used for a variety of activities. The motor is an apparatus that transforms electric energy back into mechanical energy. Some motors operate on alternating current only; other operates on direct current only. A motor that operates on both AC and DC is said to be universal. The type of current used by the motor is indicated on a tag attached to the cape of the equipment. Permanent damage may result from the use of the wrong type of current.

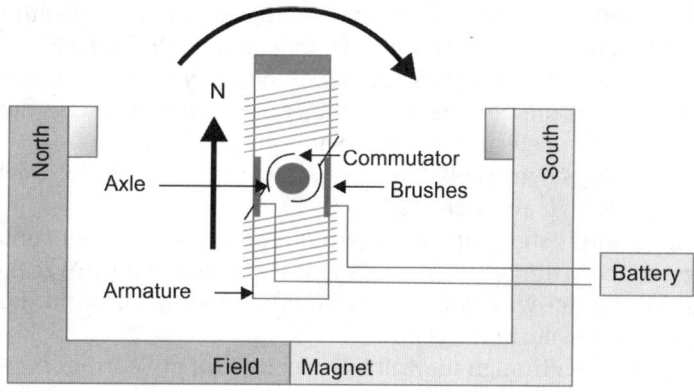

Fig. 9.15: Electric motors.

Equipment in the hospital and home should be checked for this identifying tag before use.

The Electromagnet

- The electromagnet is an example of the inter-dependability of electricity and magnetism. All electric motors are dependent upon on electromagnet for their operation **(Fig. 9.15)**.
- An electromagnet is a combination of a coil of wire and a core of iron or steel. When current passes through the wire coil, these lines of force that pass out in all directions are collected in the core where less resistance is offered them than in the surrounding air. Each molecule of the core acts like an independent magnet and combined, these form a large magnet. By using this technique, magnets with many times the strength of an ordinary magnet can be formed.
- Large electromagnets can be used to raise extremely heavy masses of iron, and still for short distances. Small electromagnets are basic in the operation of an electric bell or buzzer, telegraph equipment, telephones and other electric equipment.

■ EFFECTS OF ELECTRICITY ON THE HUMAN BODY

The study of the effects of electricity on the human body helps the health workers to take appropriate decision for appropriate action when human beings are sometimes exposed to shocks accidentally. Electric shocks may be administered therapeutically for diagnosis or for treatment of nervous and muscular disorders. The common effects are:

- The amount of electric current that flows through the body, most of the voltage is believed to cause adverse effects. The amount

of current varies directly with the voltage and inversely with the resistance between the points of application of the voltage.
- In most electric accidents contact of the body with the source of electricity is not complete and the contact resistance cuts down the amount of electric current that flows.
- Other things being equal, when contact resistance is low, flow of current is high and vice versa.
- If a person is standing on wet ground or in water so that contact resistance to the ground is low, and if at the same time he is making good contact with the source of voltage above ground, large quantities of current will flow.
- In case, even though the voltage may be low, the current may be large enough to cause death.
- When, on the other hand, contact resistance is high and the person is insulated to some degree from the ground, even though the voltage is high enough to cause a significant flow of current, heat may be generated instead, and surface burns may result.
- The central nervous system is especially susceptible to electric injury. In an electric shock, if current flow through the brain is large, unconscious may occur, retrograde amnesia is experienced and the patient remembers nothing about the accidents.
- Damage to the cranial nerves may produce sensory hallucinations.
- Blindness and deafness may result from permanent damage to the retina and organ of Corti. Death from shock is usually through the cardiac or respiratory arrest.

■ MAGNETISM

Magnetism was known to the ancient Greek tribe called the magnetes. There is evidence that magnetite or lodestone, a rock that is naturally magnetic, was known to the Greeks in the seventh century BC if not earlier. A European treatise on magnetic behavior was prepared in the thirteenth century who discussed use of lodestone in a mariner's compass. Present-day understanding of magnetic behavior arose from the combined work of many scientists in many countries. The relationship between an electric current and a magnet led Michael Faraday, to the discovery of the electromagnetic effect that is the basis of the dynamo and electric motor. Our present technology is largely built upon the many applications of electromagnetism.

Polarity

An iron or a rod of steel that has been magnetized is called a bar magnet. If such a bar magnet is suspended so that it can turn freely, it will arrange itself with its axis along a north and south line in the absence of other magnetic materials. The same end of the magnet will always turn toward the north. It is called the north-seeking or north pole of the magnet. Similarly, the other end of the magnet is called south-seeking or south pole of the magnet. Opposite poles of a magnet attract each other and similar poles repel each other.

Law of Magnetic Force

Coulomb's law: "The force of attraction or repulsion is directly proportional to the product of the strength of the poles and inversely proportional to the square of the distance between them".
The force in dynes is obtained from the following equation:

$$F = \frac{m_1 m_2}{D_2}$$

If $m_1 = m_2 = 1$ unit pole, d (distance) = 1 cm, then F = 1 dyne.

The unit pole is defined as one that exerts a force of 1 dyne upon another pole of equal strength when the two are 1cm apart in a vacuum.

Magnetic Fields

❖ The region around a magnet in which its magnetic effects are apparent is called the magnetic field of the magnet. The magnetic field may be considered to be made of many lines of force that, according to an agreement among physicists are said to pass from the north pole towards the south pole of the magnet outside the magnet.

❖ When unlike poles are brought close together, some of the lines of force pass out of the north pole of one magnet to the south pole of another magnet and two magnets are attracted **(Fig. 9.16)**.

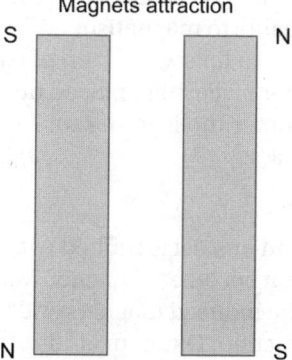

Fig. 9.16: Magnetic attraction.

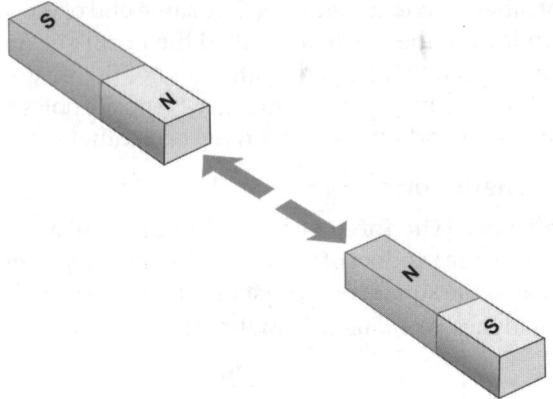

Fig. 9.17: Magnetic repulsion.

- When like poles are brought close to one another, the lines of force separate the two magnets passing from the south pole to the respective south poles of each magnet **(Fig. 9.17)**.

Field strength: "It is defined as the force in dynes acting upon a unit magnetic pole at a specified point". The unit of magnetic field strength happens to be ampere per meter or A/m. It is also represented by 'H'.

Characteristics of Magnetic Lines of Force

- When a magnet and a steel needle are separated by a piece of glass, the needle is still attracted to the magnet through the glass. Magnetic lines of force can pass through some substances such as glass, wood, zinc, lead and copper without appreciable change. Such substance are said to have low permeability to magnetism.
- When other substances such as soft iron, steel cobalt and pure nickel are placed beside a magnet, they concentrate magnetic lines of force and become magnets themselves. Such substances are said to be highly permeable to magnetism.
- Magnetic lines of force follow the path of least resistance. If a bar of soft iron and a bar of glass are placed next to the same magnet, the lines of force enter the iron because it is more perusable to magnetism than glass.

Magnetic Inductions

- When a piece of iron or steel is rubbed with a magnet or is placed in a magnetic field, it becomes a magnet. Magnets produced in the manner is said to be induced magnets and this produced is called magnetism by induction. Different kinds of iron and steel differ in their ability to retain magnetism. A very soft iron bar placed near

the magnet becomes magnetized by induction. When it is taken away from the original magnet, however, it becomes demagnetized.
- Hard steel, on the other hand, can be magnetized by induction also, but it remains magnetized which it is removed from the magnetic field.
- Substances such as iron develop the strong intensity of magnetism. When put in a magnetic field are said to be ferromagnetic. Nickel and cobalt are ferromagnetic.
- Highly magnetic alloys containing two or all three of the ferromagnetic group of metals-iron, nickel, and cobalt are important industrially. There are sometimes called permalloys because they have a high degree of permeability to magnetism.
- Other substances such as aluminum are not ferromagnetic; they are unable to concentrate lines of force in a magnetic field. These substances are weakly magnetic and are said to be paramagnetic.
- Still, other substances that are called diamagnetic tend to move away from strong magnetic fields into weaker ones.
- When a current of electricity passes through a coil of wire because the current loops act as a magnet and set up a magnetic field. If a soft iron rod is placed within the coil while the current is flowing, it becomes magnetized. The magnetic field of the current aligns the atoms in the iron rod. When the current is turned off, the atoms in the rod become disordered. A magnet made in this way is called an electromagnet.

Effect of Temperature on Magnet

- Magnetic properties of the ferromagnetic group of elements seem to be affected by temperature changes. If a bar of nickel is picked up by a magnet and heated, it will fall away from the magnet at about 350°C. Above this temperature, it is not attracted to the magnet. This is also true of iron and steel. A piece of iron will also lose its magnetic properties at a temperature above 800°C.
- It is believed that heat energy increases the internal energy of atoms and random orders of the atoms in the substance. The vigorous random motion destroys the alignment of the atoms as they exit in the magnetized state. The substance cannot exist as a magnet without the orderliness of the atoms.
- **Magnetic moment:** A useful quantity for measuring a magnetic strength is called field force (mmf).
- **Domain theory:** It is a curious fact that if a magnet is cut in two, isolated north and south poles are not produced; rather, each half becomes a complete magnet, again with north and south seeking poles. If cut in half once again four complete magnets are produced.

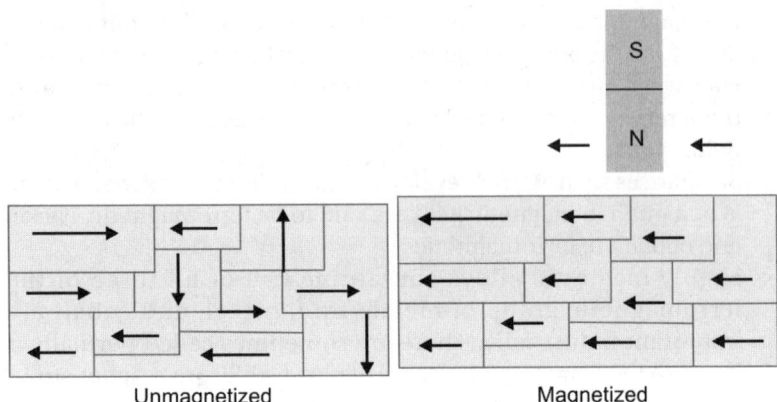
Fig. 9.18: Domain theory.

Conceivably, this subdivision could be carried down to the atomic state and each atom would become a magnet **(Fig. 9.18)**.

The domain theory of magnetism refers to a grouping of atoms with similarly aligned magnet moments into a domain. When a substance such as iron is subjected to an external magnetic field the walls of the domains move to increase the number of domains that are in line with external force. Some of the unaligned domains rotate and lineup.

Earth as a magnet: The earth itself acts as a magnet, with one magnetic pole at the north and the other almost directly opposite at the south. The magnetic field of the earth is shaped generally as if it were produced by a huge bar magnet.

■ APPLICATIONS OF THE MAGNET AND MAGNETISM

- ❖ Many devices that are important to our present civilized existence are based on magnetism. Among such devices are the telephone, telegraph, the electric bell, and the buzzer, the generation of electric current, and motors that transform the electric current into useful work **(Fig. 9.19)**.
- ❖ Magnets as such have many varied uses. In industries, they are sometimes used to remove small bites of iron or steel from grain or tobacco.
- ❖ In the hospital, a bar magnet with a rounded end may be used to remove iron and steel splinters that lodge in the conjunctiva of the eye.
- ❖ Large magnets may be used in surgery to remove foreign bodies of iron and steel from regions difficult to reach by other methods.

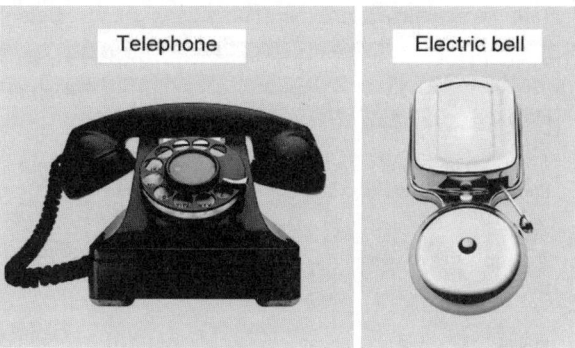

Fig. 9.19: Magnetic devices.

- A special device that has been reported operates on the basis of a magnetic force; it can be used to detect the presence of and position of metallic foreign substances in the body **(Fig. 9.19)**.
- There are reports of the passing of a catheter around eleven tortuous curves in the neck and cranium into the middle cerebral artery of the brain using a special magnetized catheter and electromagnet. The catheter is guided in the passage by gentle vibrations produced by the electromagnet on the magnet in the catheter under ordinary conditions; this is a difficult, if not possible procedure. The vibrations ease the catheter into the vessels eliminating the friction that would occur between ordinary catheters and blood vessel walls.

■ ELECTROENCEPHALOGRAPHY (EEG)

- Some action potentials within the body are manifested as surface potentials. The electroencephalogram is an example of a record of electrical activity of surface potentials that result from electrical activity within the body, in this case, the brain is the body part from where electrical activity is recorded.
- By using the electron tube amplifiers that amplify over 10 million times, it has been shown by investigators that the cerebral cortex exhibits rhythmic electric variations of potential. The potentials of the cortex are found to be present at all times except during profound anesthesia and stoppage of blood supply. When the cortex is destroyed, the pattern changes.
- Waves can be led away from the scalp by means of padded electrodes applied to the scalp or by needle electrodes placed into the scalp. One of these is a fine needle connected below the superficial layer of the scalp. Another type is a flat disk-shaped

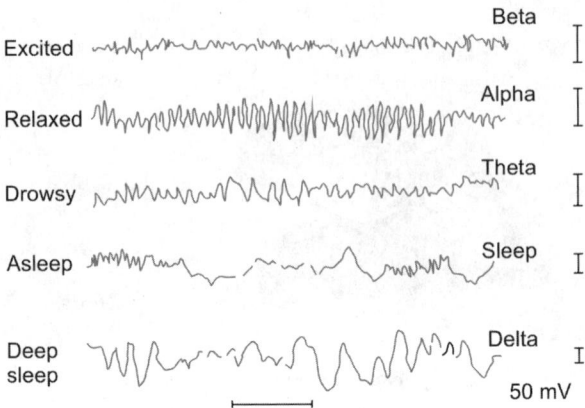
Fig. 9.20: Electroencephalogram.

electrode that is fastened to the scalp with a conducting material.
❖ The waves are the result of action potentials of the neurons of the cerebral cortex.
❖ A significant property of waves is their frequencies. The range in normal subjects to 1 to 60/sec. A crude classification is as follows **(Fig. 9.20)**:
  • **Alpha waves:** Frequency between 5 and 13/second or less
  • **β-waves (sedation):** 14 to 60/second.
  • **Delta waves (sedation):** 5/sec or less.

Classification according to form of wave:
❖ Spiked
❖ Flattened
❖ Serrated

A recording is done graphically or electrically by a cathode ray recording. The recording is called an electroencephalogram (EEG). The waves are evaluated according to their frequencies, voltages, incidences, waveforms and patterns.

Uses of EEG

❖ In diagnosing epilepsy, tumors, hematoma, trauma, drug addiction, and alcoholism.
❖ Studies have been made that show that the depth of anesthesia experienced by a patient may be revealed by encephalography.
❖ In one study, seven levels of brain depression from the normal waking state to a complete absence of electric discharges have been described for ether.

■ ELECTROCARDIOGRAPHY (ECG)

- ❖ In this case, a record of surface potentials is made of active heart muscles during the cardiac cycle.
- ❖ Several methods are employed today to record ECG.

Process of ECG

Generally, electric charges are carried from the surface of the body to a fine gold-plated quartz fiber. That is supported between the poles of an electromagnet. As current passes through the fiber, it moves, a beam of light that passes across the poles of a magnet and the image of the motion of the fiber is recorded on a film.

In another method, a heated stylus is attached to the moving fiber and the stylus describes the pattern of the electrical activity of the heart on a roll of plastic-coated paper.

Technique

In the technique, generally used, electrodes are placed on the right arm, left arm, and left leg. Other electrodes are placed at various levels of the chest and back. Any two of these electrodes may be connected to a galvanometer at any one time and the voltage of one of them with respect to the other one is recorded. These voltages will be the algebraic sum of the body surface voltages under each the electrodes. The voltages are associated with electrical manifestations of the activities in the cardiac cycle. During the cardiac cycle, when the upper part of the heart is active, the upper extremities will be at a lower electric potential than the lower extremities. The difference in potential is small, but it can be amplified by a triode tube.

During a recording of ECG, the body acts as a container of saline solution, which is a conductor. The recording electrodes that are fixed to the skin with a conducting paste respond to the potential field produced by heart action.

Wave Pattern

ECG represents a series of waves and deflections during a complete cycle. The waves are known as the P wave, QRS complex, and the T wave **(Fig. 9.21)**.

- ❖ **P wave:** Follows the initiation of a heartbeat by a pacemaker. The wave is produced by the movement of a wave of electrical activity through the atria. This represents the atrial contraction. It represents the electrical activities associated with the spread of the original impulse from the sinoatrial node (SA) through the atria. If the P waves were absent or altered, the cardiac impulse originates outside the SA node.

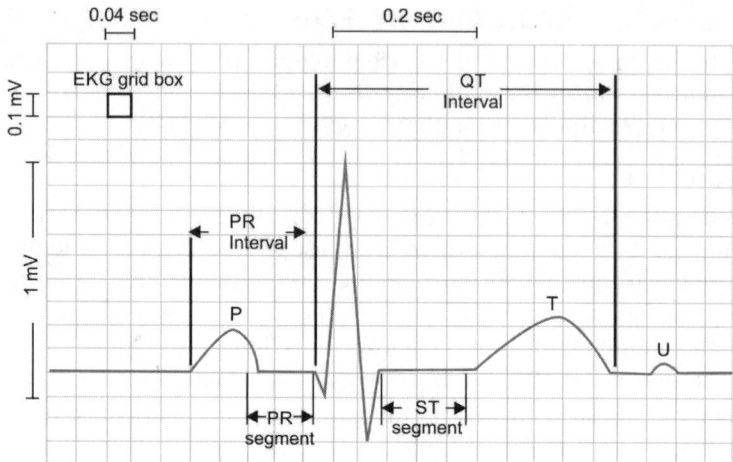

Fig. 9.21: Electrocardiogram.

- ❖ **PR interval:** This represents the time required for the impulse to travel from the SA node to the atrioventricular node. If this interval is prolonged, a conduction delay exists in the AV node (e.g., first-degree heart block). If the PR interval is shortened; the impulse must have reached the ventricle through a "shortcut." (as in Wolff-Parkinson-White syndrome).
- ❖ **QRS complex:** This represents ventricular electrical depolarization associated with ventricular contraction. This complex consists of an initial downward (negative) deflection (Q) wave, a large upward (positive) deflection (R wave) and a small downwards deflection (S wave). A widened QRS complex indicates abnormal or prolonged ventricular depolarization (as in bundle branch block).
- ❖ **ST-segment:** This represents the period between the completion of depolarization and the beginning of repolarization of the ventricular muscles. This segment may be elevated or depressed in transient muscle ischemia (e.g., angina) or 'a muscle injury', as in the early stages of myocardial infarction.
- ❖ **T wave:** This represents ventricular repolarization (i.e., return to neutral electrical activity).
- ❖ **U wave:** This deflection follows the T wave and is usually quite small. It represents the repolarization of the Purkinje fibers within the ventricular. Through the analysis of these, waveforms and time intervals, valuable information about the heart may be obtained.

■ PHONOCARDIOGRAPHY

The phonocardiography records the sounds of the heart by means of suction microphones that are attached to the chest wall.

The pressure waves produced by the sound are connected to electric current, amplified, and recorded in a similar manner to the way in which the electrical impulses are recorded on ECG. In some cases, the electrical impulses are reconverted to sound that can be recorded or heard directly.

■ ELECTROMYOGRAPHY (EMG)

Electromyography is a study of the electrical activity of the muscle to determine the condition of the muscle and its nerve supply either in a particular disease or following injury. The electrical activity is picked up by needle electrodes that are inserted into the muscle. The needle is insulated except for the tip; consequently, it detects only electric variations in the region of the tip. The electrode voltage is amplified and can be observed directly on the screen of the cathode rays oscilloscope. If a permanent record is desired, the visual image of electric changes that appear on the screen may be photographed. The amplified voltage may also be transmitted to the loudspeaker and heard.

■ ELECTROMYOGRAPHY PATTERN

❖ There is a definite EMG pattern for normal contracting muscle. Differences obtained from the normal pattern are interpreted.
❖ Amplitudes of EMG potential vary in parts of a muscle. Observations are usually made in several parts of the muscle in order to get a representative (**Fig. 9.22**).

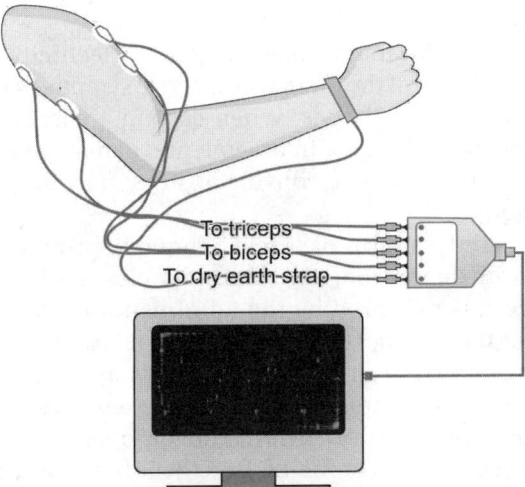

Fig. 9.22: Electromyography.

- There are also difficulties of patterns among different muscle. The uterus during labor was the subject of one electromyographic study.
- In addition to records of surface potentials related to action potential, some studies have been made of potential gradients during the formation of neoplasm and peripheral lesions, wound healing and the menstrual cycle.

■ ELECTROSTIMULATION

Some investigators believe that galvanic stimulation of denervated muscle may help to preserve muscle tissue and prevent atrophy. In fact, galvanic stimulators have been used in treating some patients. The apparatus consists of two small cathodes that are placed on either end of the affected muscle. A small galvanic current generator is connected to a dry cell and the time and the strength of the current are regulated by a stimulator that can be placed in the pocket of the patients where it is easily accessible to him. The patients control the stimulation by a special device on the apparatus.

In addition to artificial muscle stimulation; electrotherapy includes the use of direct current and the application of high frequency current. There have been reports of electrical stimulation of the phrenic nerves to induce respiration.

■ ELECTROCONVULSIVE THERAPY (ECT)

- ECT is a physical or somatic therapy in which, with the help of two electrodes current is passed through the temporal region in between the two hemispheres of the brain to produce grandmal seizures.
- It has been shown that a small current of electricity applied to areas of the cortex of the brain will produce symptoms manifested as simple muscle twitches. When certain areas, described as epileptogenic areas, exist in an epileptic patient, stimulation of these areas will produce convulsions that may be localized or generalized.
- ECT is a painless form of electric therapy, primarily used for patients with depression, and schizophrenic disorders.
- The patient is prepared by the administration of barbiturate anesthesia and an injection of a chemical relaxant.
- An electric current of 70 to 130 volts is applied for 0.1 to 1 second through electrodes placed on the temporal region. This immediately produces seizures or convulsions **(Fig. 9.23)**.
- The biological effects of the ECT are believed to be achieved by neurophysiological, neuroendocrine and neurochemical changes.

CHAPTER 9: Electricity and Electromagnetism

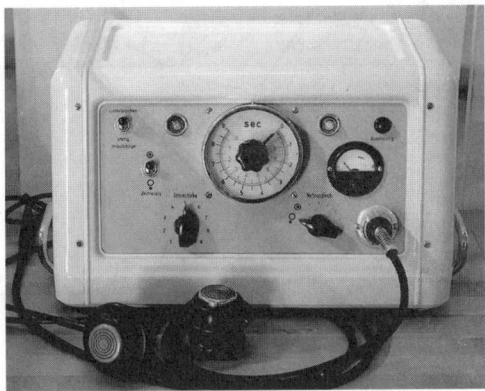

Fig. 9.23: Electroconvulsive therapy machine.

However, the catecholamine hypothesis of its mechanism of action is more widely accepted.
- There is no absolute contraindication of ECT. However, it had increased risk in patients with increased intracranial pressure either due to brain tumor, hematoma, hemorrhage, osteoporosis or recent history of fracture or thrombolytic therapy.

■ ELECTRONIC CARDIAC PACEMAKER
- A device called the electronic cardiac pacemaker maintains normal heartbeats in cases of heart block or arrhythmia that prevents normal transmission of impulses from SA-mode, the natural cardiac pacemaker.
- An electronic cardiac pacemaker may be temporary or permanent.
- Temporary pacemakers are helpful to persons who have a transient blockage of the conduction pathway after a myocardial infarction or cardiac surgery. If the chest wall is opened as during surgery pacing electrodes may be implanted on the epicardium, extended through the chest incision, and connected to an external pacing battery control box. A pacing electrode can also be implanted directly into the right ventricle by passing it through the external jugular subclavian antecubital or femoral vein. In this case, to the electrodes may then be connected to the pacing battery box that is kept near the patient. The temporary pacer is usually tried first with most patients because the device can be removed when necessary relatively simple. In addition, battery can be replaced early if required **(Fig. 9.24)**.
- In cases of irreversible cardiac damage and complete conductive pathway blockage, a permanent pacemaker may be used.

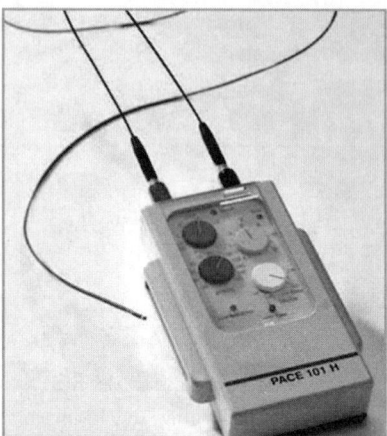

Fig. 9.24: External cardiac pacemaker.

The electrode can be implanted through the vein as a temporary one, but here battery box about the size of a pocket watch a smaller is permanently implanted into the subcutaneous tissue of the chest wall or abdomen. These batteries may be of several types of different life expectancies.
- In the types, these pacemakers could be fixed or demand in the input of electric impulses.

■ BRAIN PACEMAKER
- A device consisting of a plate of silicon-covered dacron mesh that contains four pairs of platinum disk electrodes, an internally implanted radio frequency receiver and a pocket-sized external transmitter have been reported beneficial to patients with uncontrolled seizures and spasticity associated with epilepsy, stroke, cerebral palsy and other brain disorders (**Fig. 9.25**).
- The plates are applied to the cerebellar surface through small occipital and suboccipital craniotomies. Two receivers are implanted in the chest below the clavicles and are connected by subcutaneous leads to the plates. An antenna is placed directly over the receiver and stimulation is controlled by an external transmitter.
- The rationale briefly is that stimulating the cerebellar cortex is inhibitory and assists with the control of skeletal activity. The stimulator contains an automatic timer. The rate, frequency, and timing depends on the person's requirement. Generally, the electrodes in each plate are stimulated simultaneously several minutes off the several minutes on.

CHAPTER 9: Electricity and Electromagnetism

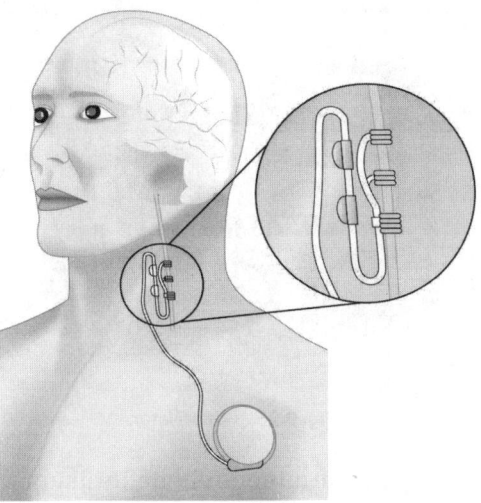

Fig. 9.25: Brain pacemaker.

- A button located in the transmitter that is activated simultaneously rather than alternate stimulation is reported to be successful in preventing or aborting seizures. This technique is still experimental, but if perfected, offers a means for normal life to a person who might otherwise be seriously limited.

■ DEFIBRILLATION

Cardiac defibrillation is the act of administering a transthoracic electrical current to a person experiencing one of the two lethal ventricular dysrhythmias, ventricular fibrillation (VF) or pulseless ventricular tachycardia (VT). A defibrillator is an electric device used to deliver an electrical current (shock) of present voltage to the heart through paddles placed on the chest wall (closed-chest procedure). This current causes the entire myocardium to depolarize completely at the moment of shock, thus producing transient asystole and allowing the heart's intrinsic pacemaker to regain control. The amount of energy required to produce this effect is determined largely by the client's transthoracic impedance or resistance to current flow. Because of this factor, the amount of energy that reaches the heart is less than the amount that the defibrillator is charged to deliver **(Fig. 9.26)**.

The procedure is associated with potential hazards, particularly myocardial damage. The higher the amount of energy or frequency of the shock, the greater the risk of injury. Advances in the equipment now allow measurement of transthoracic impedance.

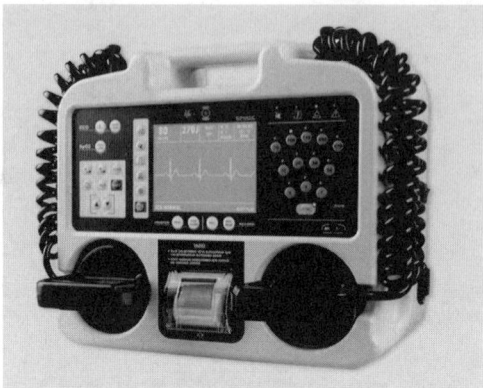

Fig. 9.26: Defibrillator.

Once impedance is determined, the defibrillator automatically selects the amount of the current. It is expected this mode of defibrillation will reduce the risk of complications.

The degree of transthoracic resistance depends on several variables:
* **Energy level:** The higher the energy level that is selected, the more current will follow. Usually, 360 J with monophasic and 200 J with biphasic is delivered during defibrillation.
* **Number and frequency of shock:** The more shocks administrated and the shorter the time between them, the lower the transthoracic resistance.
* **Ventilation phase:** Resistance is lower when there is less air (and therefore a smaller diameter) in the lungs.
* **Paddle size:** The larger the paddle, the lower the resistance.
* **Chest size:** The smaller the distance between the defibrillator electrodes once they are in place, the lower the resistance.
* **Paddle-skin interface material:** Conductive material between the skin and paddle, helping to overcome transthoracic resistance. Exerts, about 25 pounds of pressure on each paddle.
* **Paddle placement:** Place one paddle on the upper chest, to the right of the sternum; place the other paddle on the lower left chest, to the left of the nipple, with the center of the paddle in the midaxillary line. If the client has a permanent pacemaker or internal cardiac defibrillation, place the paddles at least 5 inches away from the generator to avoid damaging it. If a temporary pacing system is in use, disconnect the pacing lead from the pulse generator immediately before defibrillation and reconnect it after the shock.

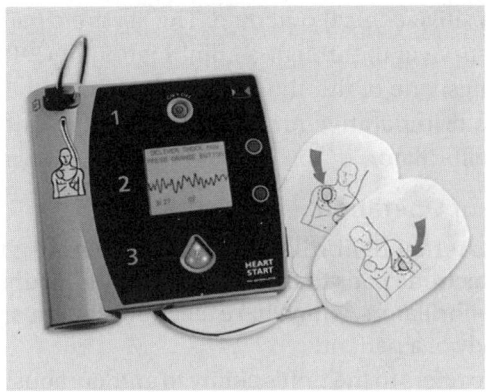

Fig. 9.27: Automated external defibrillator.

■ AUTOMATED EXTERNAL DEFIBRILLATOR

An automated external defibrillator (AED) is a portable electronic device **(Fig. 9.27)** that automatically diagnoses the potentially life-threatening cardiac arrhythmias of ventricular fibrillation and ventricular tachycardia in a patient, and is able to treat them through defibrillation, the application of electrical therapy which stops the arrhythmia, allowing the heart to reestablish an effective rhythm. AEDs are designed to be simple to use for the layman, and the use of AEDs is taught in many first aid, first responder, and basic life support (BLS) level CPR classes.

Uses

An automated external defibrillator is used in cases of life-threatening cardiac arrhythmias which lead to cardiac arrest. The rhythms that the device will treat are usually limited to:
- Pulseless ventricular tachycardia (shortened to VT or V-tach)
- Ventricular fibrillation (shortened to VF or V-fib)

In each of these two types of shockable cardiac arrhythmia, the heart is active, but in a life-threatening, dysfunctional pattern. In ventricular tachycardia, the heart beats too fast to effectively pump blood. Ultimately, ventricular tachycardia leads to ventricular fibrillation. In ventricular fibrillation, the electrical activity of the heart becomes chaotic, preventing the ventricle from effectively pumping blood. The fibrillation in the heart decreases over time, and will eventually reach asystole.

Automated external defibrillators (AEDs), like all defibrillators, are not designed to shock asystole ('flat line' patterns) as this will not have a positive clinical outcome. The asystolic patient only has a chance of survival if, through a combination of CPR and cardiac stimulant drugs, one of the shockable rhythms can be established, which makes it imperative for CPR to be carried out prior to the arrival of a defibrillator.

Mechanism of Operation

Automated external defibrillator is external because the operator applies the electrode pads to the bare chest of the victim, as opposed to internal defibrillators, which have electrodes surgically implanted inside the body of a patient.

Automatic refers to the unit's ability to autonomously analyze the patient's condition, and to assist this, the vast majority of units have spoken prompts, and some may also have visual displays to instruct the user. When turned on or opened, the AED will instruct the user to connect the electrodes (pads) to the patient. Once the pads are attached, everyone should avoid touching the patient so as to avoid false readings by the unit. The pads allow the AED to examine the electrical output from the heart and determine if the patient is in a shockable rhythm (either ventricular fibrillation or ventricular tachycardia). If the device determines that a shock is warranted, it will use the battery to charge its internal capacitor in preparation to deliver the shock. This system is not only safer (charging only when required), but also allows for faster delivery of the electrical current.

When charged, the device instructs the user to ensure no one is touching the victim and then to press a button to deliver the shock; human intervention is usually required to deliver the shock to the patient in order to avoid the possibility of accidental injury to another person (which can result from a responder or bystander touching the patient at the time of the shock). Depending on the manufacturer and particular model, after the shock is delivered most devices will analyze the victim and either instruct that CPR be given, or administer another shock.

Many AED units have an 'event memory' which stores the ECG of the patient along with details of the time the unit was activated and the number and strength of any shocks delivered. Some units also have voice recording abilities to monitor the actions taken by the personnel in order to ascertain if these had any impact on the survival outcome. All this recorded data can be either downloaded to a computer or printed out so that the providing organization or responsible body is able to see the effectiveness of both CPR and defibrillation.

Automated external defibrillators (AEDs) available to the public may be semi-automatic or fully automatic. Fully automatic units are likely to have a few buttons, often activating as soon as the case is opened, and possibly just one button to shock, or in some cases, this will be performed automatically. The user has no input in the operation of the unit apart from attaching the pads and following the prompts. Health care professionals and other trained responders may use a semi-automatic defibrillator, which is likely to have an ECG readout display, and the possibility to override the rhythm analysis software. This allows trained personnel to provide a higher level of care.

The first commercially available AEDs were all of a monophasic type, which gave a high-energy shock, up to 360–4400 joules depending on the model. This caused increased cardiac injury and in some cases second and third-degree burns around the shock pad sites. Newer AEDs (manufactured after late 2003) have tended to utilize biphasic algorithms which give two sequential lower-energy shocks of 120–200 joules, with each shock moving in an opposite polarity between the pads. This lower-energy waveform has proven more effective in clinical tests, as well as offering a reduced rate of complications and reduced recovery time.

■ MAGNETIC RESONANCE IMAGING (MRI)

Magnetic resonance imaging (MRI), or nuclear magnetic resonance imaging (NMRI), is primarily a medical imaging technique most commonly used in radiology to visualize detailed internal structure and limited function of the body. MRI provides much greater contrast between the different soft tissues of the body than computed tomography (CT) does, making it especially useful in neurological (brain), musculoskeletal, cardiovascular, and oncological (cancer) imaging. Unlike CT, it uses no ionizing radiation but uses a powerful magnetic field to align the nuclear magnetization of (usually) hydrogen atoms in water in the body. Radiofrequency (RF) fields are used to systematically alter the alignment of this magnetization, causing the hydrogen nuclei to produce a rotating magnetic field detectable by the scanner. This signal can be manipulated by additional magnetic fields to build up enough information to construct an image of the body **(Fig. 9.28)**.

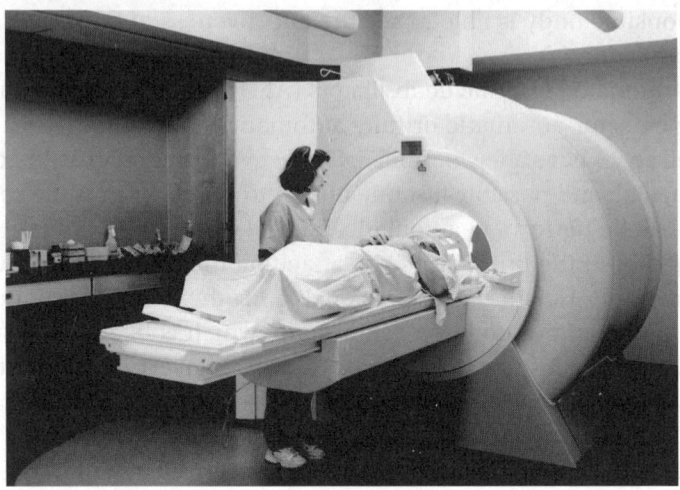

Fig. 9.28: Magnetic resonance imaging.

Mechanism of Operation and Uses

The body is largely composed of water molecules which each contain two hydrogen nuclei or protons. When a person goes inside the powerful magnetic field of the scanner, the magnetic moments of these protons align with the direction of the field.

A radiofrequency electromagnetic field is then briefly turned on, causing the protons to alter their alignment relative to the field. When this field is turned off, the protons return to the original magnetization alignment. These alignment changes create a signal which can be detected by the scanner. The frequency at which the protons resonate depends on the strength of the magnetic field. The position of protons in the body can be determined by applying additional magnetic fields during the scan which allows an image of the body to be built up. These are created by turning gradients coils on and off which creates the knocking sounds heard during an MR scan.

Diseased tissue, such as tumors, can be detected because the protons in different tissues return to their equilibrium state at different rates. By changing the parameters on the scanner this effect is used to create contrast between different types of body tissue.

Contrast agents may be injected intravenously to enhance the appearance of blood vessels, tumors, or inflammation. Contrast agents may also be directly injected into a joint in the case of arthrograms, and MR images of joints. Unlike CT, MRI uses no ionizing radiation and is generally a very safe procedure. Patients with some metal implants, cochlear implants, and cardiac pacemakers are prevented from having an MRI scan due to the effects of the strong magnetic field and powerful radiofrequency pulses.

MRI is used to image every part of the body, and is particularly useful for neurological conditions, disorders of the muscles and joints, for evaluating tumors, and for showing abnormalities in the heart and blood vessels.

■ CAT SCAN

The word "tomography" is derived from the Greek tomos (slice) and graphein (to write). Computed tomography was originally known as the "EMI scan". It was later known as computed axial tomography (CAT or CT scan) and body section roentgenography. Computed tomography (CT) is a medical imaging method employing tomography created by computer processing. Digital geometry processing is used to generate a three-dimensional image of the inside of an object from a large series of two-dimensional X-ray images taken around a single axis of rotation. The machine was developed by physicist Allan MacLeod Cormack and electrical engineer Godfrey Hounsfield.

The CT scan is essentially an X-ray study, wherein a series of rays are rotated around a specified body part, and computer-generated cross-sectional images are produced. The advantage of these tomographic images compared to conventional X-rays is that they contain detailed information about a specified area in cross-section, eliminating the superimposition of images, which provides a tremendous advantage over plain films. CT scans provide excellent clinicopathological correlation for a suspected illness.

- ❖ **Uses:** It is used to diagnose several disorders of a different area of the body:
  - **Head:** CT scanning of the head is typically used to detect:
    - Bleeding, brain injury, and skull fractures
    - Bleeding due to a ruptured/leaking aneurysm in a patient with a sudden severe headache
    - A blood clot or bleeding within the brain shortly after a patient exhibits symptoms of a stroke
  - A stroke
    - Brain tumors
    - Enlarged brain cavities in patients with hydrocephalus
    - Diseases/malformations of the skull

- **Chest:** CT can be used for detecting both acute and chronic changes in the lung parenchyma, that is, the internals of the lungs. Like emphysema, fibrosis, lung cancer, pneumonia, etc. CT angiography of the chest may be helpful in the detection of pulmonary embolism (PE) and aortic dissection.
- **Abdominal and pelvic:** CT is a sensitive method for diagnosis of abdominal diseases, especially cancer; can also be helpful in the investigation of abdominal pain to rule out renal stones, appendicitis, pancreatitis, diverticulitis, abdominal aortic aneurysm, and bowel obstruction, etc.

Process

X-ray slice data is generated using an X-ray source that rotates around the object; X-ray sensors are positioned on the opposite side of the circle from the X-ray source. The earliest sensors were scintillation detectors, with photomultiplier tubes excited by (typically) cesium iodide crystals. Cesium iodide was replaced during the eighties by ion chambers containing high-pressure xenon gas. These systems were in turn replaced by scintillation systems based on photodiodes instead of photomultipliers and modern scintillation materials with more desirable characteristics. Many data scans are progressively taken as the object is gradually passed through the gantry. They are combined together by mathematical procedures known as tomographic reconstruction. The data are arranged in a matrix in memory, and each data point is convolved with its neighbors, according to a seed algorithm using Fast Fourier Transform techniques. This dramatically increases the resolution of each voxel (volume element). Then a process is known as back projection essentially reverses the acquisition geometry and stores the result in another memory array. This data can then be displayed, photographed, or used as input for further processing, such as multiplanar reconstruction.

In conventional CT machines, an X-ray tube and detector are physically rotated behind a circular shroud (see the image above right); in the electron beam tomography (EBT) the tube is far larger and has higher power to support the high temporal resolution. The electron beam is deflected in a hollow funnel-shaped vacuum chamber. X-rays are generated when the beam hits the stationary target. The detector is also stationary. This arrangement can result in very fast scans, but is extremely expensive.

The data stream representing the varying radiographic intensity is sensed at the detectors on the opposite side of the circle during each sweep, then computer processes to calculate cross-sectional

CHAPTER 9: Electricity and Electromagnetism

estimations of the radiographic density, expressed in Hounsfield units. Sweeps cover 360° or just over 180° in conventional machines, and 220° in EBT.

Newer machines with faster computer systems and newer software strategies can process not only individual cross-sections, but continuously change cross-sections ions as the gantry, with the object to be imaged, is slowly and smoothly slid through the X-ray circle. These are called helical or spiral CT machines. Their computer systems integrate the data of the moving individual slices to generate three-dimensional volumetric information (3D-CT scan), in turn, viewable from multiple different perspectives on attached CT workstation monitors. This type of data acquisition requires enormous processing power, as the data is arriving in a continuous stream and must be processed in real-time.

■ QUESTIONS

Q.1: The electronic device that picks up sound waves and converts them into electric current is called.............
Q.2: The process in which electric shock is imparted to the chest to normalize heartbeat is called...............
Q.3: Electric switches should not be touched with wet hands.
Q.4: Therapeutic uses of electricity.
Q.5: Why synthetic cloth dresses are not allowed in operation theaters?
Q.6: Why the use of three-pin plugs in electrical connection safe than two-pin plugs?
Q.7: Use of silk or nylon is generally forbidden in operating theaters. Explain
Q.8: Human body is a good conductor of electricity. Discuss

■ BIBLIOGRAPHY

1. American Red Cross. CPR/AED for the Professional Rescuer (participant's manual). Yardley, PA: StayWell, 2006.
2. Bird J. Electrical and Electronic Principles and Technology, 3rd edition, Newnes, 2007.
3. Bullock TH. Electroreception, Springer, 2005.
4. Close F. The New Cosmic Onion: Quarks and the Nature of the Universe, CRC Press, 2007.
5. Dibner B. Oersted and the Discovery of Electromagnetism. Blaisdell Publishing Company, 1961.

6. Dosdall DJ, Fast VG, Ideker RE. Mechanisms of defibrillation. Annu Rev Biomed Eng. 2010;12:233–258. doi:10.1146/annurev-bioeng-070909-105305
7. Duffin WJ. Electricity and Magnetism, 3rd edition, McGraw-Hill, 1980.
8. Goyal A, Chhabra L, Sciammarella JC, et al. Defibrillation. [Updated 2022 Feb 7]. In: StatPearls [Internet]. Treasure Island (FL): StatPearls Publishing; 2022 Jan-. Available from: https://www.ncbi.nlm.nih.gov/books/NBK499899/
9. Griffiths DJ. Introduction to Electrodynamics, 3rd edition. Prentice Hall, 1998.
10. Hammond P. Electromagnetism for Engineers, Pergamon, 1981.
11. Jackson JD. Classical Electrodynamics, 3rd edition. Wiley, 1998.
12. Morley A, Hughes E. Principles of Electricity, 5th edition, Longman, 1994.
13. Morris SC. Life's Solution: Inevitable Humans in a Lonely Universe, Cambridge University Press, 2003.
14. Naidu MS, Kamataru V. High Voltage Engineering, Tata McGraw-Hill, 1982. Nilsson, James; Riedel, Susan. Electric Circuits, Prentice Hall, 2007.
15. Patel PR, De Jesus O. CT Scan. [Updated 2022 Jan 5]. In: StatPearls [Internet]. Treasure Island (FL): StatPearls Publishing; 2022 Jan-. Available from: https://www.ncbi.nlm.nih.gov/books/NBK567796/
16. Patterson WC. Transforming Electricity: The Coming Generation of Change, Earthscan, 1999.
17. Rothwell EJ, Cloud MJ. Electromagnetics. CRC Press, 2001.
18. Sears F, et. al., University Physics, Sixth Edition, Addison Wesley, 1982. Benjamin, P. A history of electricity (the intellectual rise in electricity) from antiquity to the days of Benjamin Franklin. New York: J. Wiley and Sons. 1998.
19. Simpson B. Electrical Stimulation and the Relief of Pain, Elsevier Health Sciences, 2003.
20. Stewart J. Intermediate Electromagnetic Theory, World Scientific, 2001.
21. Tipler P. Physics for Scientists and Engineers: Vol. 2: Light, Electricity and Magnetism, 4th edition. WH Freeman. 1998.
22. Udupa JK, Herman GT. 3D Imaging in Medicine, 2nd edition, CRC Press, 2000.
23. Wangsness RK, Cloud MJ. Electromagnetic Fields, 2nd Edition, Wiley, 1986.

CHAPTER 10

Nuclear Physics

Suresh K Sharma, Navjot Kaur

Chapter Outline

- Structure of Atom
- Applications
- Clinical Uses of Radioisotopes and Radio Elements
- Radiation Protection Limits
- Instruments Used for Detection of Ionizing Radiation, X-rays

■ INTRODUCTION

You might have exposure to the model of the atom since your school education. The atom can be visualized as a mini solar system in which the nucleus is surrounded by electrons. You may also be aware that the atomic nucleus is a very small and dense object consisting of two types of particles namely proton and neutron. It has taken a long time and a series of classic experiments from the early ideas about atoms to the present-day atomic models.

Nuclear physics is the study of the protons and neutrons at the center of an atom and the interactions that hold them together in a space just a few femtometers across. For example, nuclear reactions include radioactive decay, fission, the break-up of a nucleus, and fusion, the merging of nuclei.

■ STRUCTURE OF ATOM

Thomson's Atomic Model

After the discovery of electrons and protons, the scientists started thinking of arranging these particles in an atom. The first simple model was proposed by JJ Thomson known as Thomson's Atomic model. JJ Thomson proposed that the positive charge is spread over a sphere in which electrons are embedded to make the atom as a whole neutral.

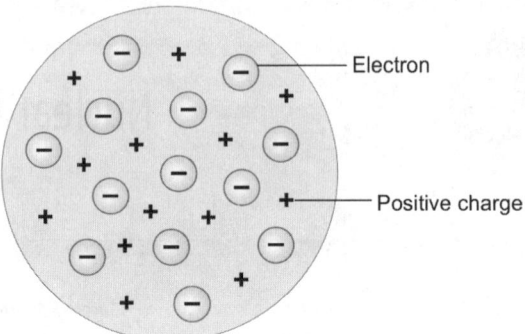

Thomson's plum pudding model

Fig. 10.1: Thomson's atomic model.

The radius of the sphere is of the order of 10-p10 cm, which is equal to the size of the atom. This model was much like raisins in a pudding and is also known as the Thomson plum pudding model. The model could explain why only negatively charged particles are emitted when a metal is heated and never the positively charged particles. It also could explain how the ions and ionic compounds of chemistry are formed **(Fig. 10.1)**.

Rutherford's Model of an Atom

Thomson's model had some advantages and could explain a few phenomena successfully, but at the same time, it had certain disadvantages too. According to this model, charges are spread over the total volume of the atom, but this was not consistent with the fact that cathode rays pass through the atom almost freely. The atom must have a lot of space for this to happen.

Rutherford did an experiment known as Rutherford's scattering experiment. In this experiment, a piece of a radioactive substance is placed in a lead block. The block is constructed in such a way with slits that only a narrow beam of X-particles could escape. The beam of alpha particles then passes through the thin gold foil to detect alpha particles after scattering, a movable circular screen coated with zinc sulfate is placed around a gold foil **(Fig. 10.2)**.

The following observations were made from these experiments:
- Most of the α-particles nearly pass through the gold foil undetected. It means there must be a very large empty space.
- Some of them get deflected from some angles. It means there is a heavy positively charged mass present in the atom.

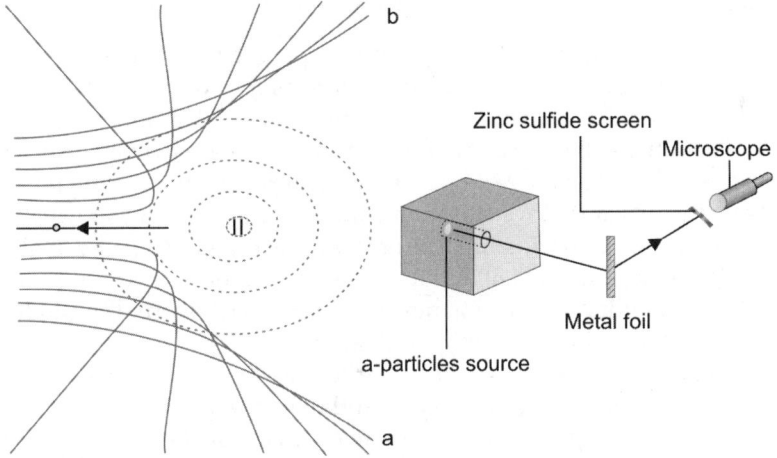

Fig. 10.2: Rutherford's scattering experiment.

Moreover, this mass must be occupying a very small space within the atom because only a few particles suffered large deflections.

❖ Very few, about one in 20,000 did not pass through the foil at all but suffered large deflections (more than 90%) or even came back suffering a deflection of 180°. It means there is a direct collision with the heavy positively charged mass.

Main Features

❖ In an atom, the entire mass and the positive charge are concentrated in a very small region at the center known as the nucleus.
❖ The positive charge of the nucleus is due to protons.
❖ The mass of the nucleus is due to protons and some other neutral particles each having a mass nearly equal to the mass of the proton. It was called a neutron.
❖ The nucleus is surrounded by negatively charged electrons which balance the positive charge on the nucleus. Thus, the atom is electrically neutral.
❖ The electrons are not stationary but are revolving around the nucleus at very high speeds like planets revolving around the sun. Thus, electrons are planetary electrons.
❖ The electrons and nucleus are held together by electrostatic forces of attraction.
❖ Most of the space in an atom between the nucleus and revolving electrons is empty.

Failures

- It was shown by Clark Maxwell that a charged body moving under the influence of attractive forces loses energy continuously in the form of electromagnetic radiations. Thus, unlike a planet, the electron is a charged body, it should emit radiations while revolving around the nucleus. As a result, the electron should lose energy at every turn and move closer and closer to the nucleus following a spiral path. Consequently, the orbit will become smaller and finally the electron would fall into the nucleus. In other words, the atom should collapse, but this never happens. Therefore, the model cannot explain the stability of an atom.
- This model does not explain the structure of atoms, i.e. distribution of electrons around the nucleus and their energies.
- It does not explain the appearance of many spectral lines of the hydrogen atom.

Bohr's Model of an Atom

- An atom consists of a small heavy positively charged nucleus in the center surrounded by electrons. The electrons in an atom revolve around the nucleus only in certain selected circular paths called orbits. These orbits are associated with definite energies and are called energy shells or energy levels. These are numbered as 1, 2, 3, 4, etc. from the nucleus. These are alternatively designated as K, L, M, N, shells, etc. **(Fig. 10.3)**.
- As long as the electrons remain in a particular path, it does not lose or gain energy. This means that the energy of electrons in a

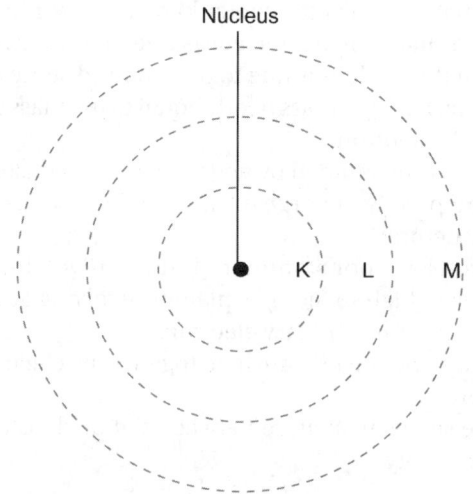

Fig. 10.3: Orbits of an atom.

particular energy shell remains constant. Therefore, these orbits are also called stationary states. The term stationary does not mean that electron is stationary, but it means that the energy of the electron does not change with time. This accounts for the stability of an atom.
- Only those orbits are permitted in which the angular momentum of the electron is a whole number multiple of h/2π (where h is Planck's constant). An electron like any other moving body in a circular orbit has an angular momentum equal to mvr. Thus, according to Bohr, the angular momentum mvr is a whole number multiple of h/2π.

$$mvr = \frac{nh}{2\pi}$$

where, $n = 1, 2, 3...$

- The energy is emitted or absorbed only when electrons jump from one energy level to another. When energy is supplied to an atom, its electrons absorb one or more quantum of energy and jump to a higher energy level. This higher energy state of the electron is called its excited state. When the electron jumps back to the lower energy level, it radiates the same energy. The amount of energy emitted or absorbed is given by the difference in the energies of the two energy levels concerned. That is:

$\Delta E = E_2 - E_1$

$E_2 - E_1$

$E_1 - E_2$

Energy absorbed Energy released

Success

- Bohr's atomic model the stability of an atom. According to Bohr, an electron revolving in a particular orbit cannot lose energy. Therefore, emission of radiation is not possible as long as the electron remains at one of its energy levels, and hence, there is no cause of instability in his model.
- Bohr's concept of atoms explained successfully the atomic spectrum of the hydrogen atom. From Bohr's atomic model, it is clear that electrons can have only a certain definite energy levels. When the electron is present as close to the nucleus as possible, the atom has the minimum possible energy and is said to be in the ground state. When energy from some outside source is supplied, it jumps to a higher energy state. This is called the excited state. This excited state is unstable the electrons come back to lower energy levels and energy is emitted in the form of a quantum equal to the difference in energy between the two levels. When this quantum

of energy strikes the photographic plate, it gives its impression in the form of a line.

Now:
$$E_2 - E_1 = h\nu$$
$$\nu = E_2 - E_1/h$$

Since
$$\nu = \text{frequency} = c/\lambda$$
$$c/\lambda = E_2 - E_1/h$$
$$\lambda = hc/E_2 - E_1$$

Since h and c are constants and $E_2 - E_1$ corresponds to definite energy, thus each transition from one level to another will produce light of a definite wavelength. This is observed as a line in the spectrum of the hydrogen atom. If the electron jumps from third to first energy level, then:
$$\lambda' = hc/E_3 - E_1$$

Similarly,
$$\lambda'' = hc/E_4 - E_1 \quad \text{and} \quad \lambda''' = hc/E_5 - E_1$$

Thus different spectral lines in the spectra of atoms correspond to different transitions of electrons from higher energy levels to lower energy levels **(Fig. 10.4)**.

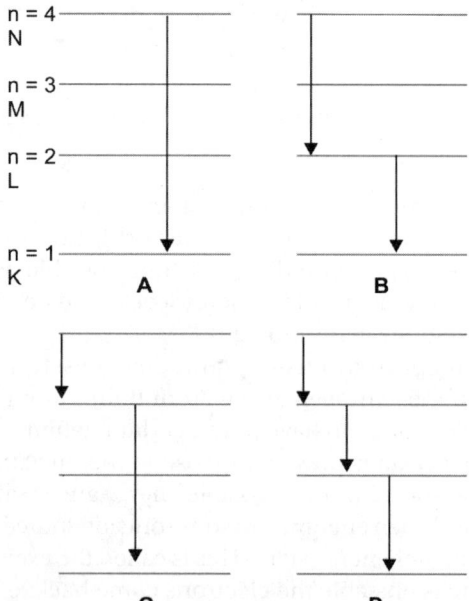

Fig. 10.4 A to D: Simultaneous appearance of a large number of lines in the spectrum of hydrogen.

In any sample of hydrogen gas, there are a large number of hydrogen atoms. When energy is supplied by passing electric discharge, the electrons in different atoms absorb different amounts of energy, therefore, they are raised to different energy states. For example, the electrons in some atoms may jump to the second energy level (L) while in others may be raised to third (M), fourth (N), and fifth (O) energy levels, and so on. Now the excited electrons come back from the higher energy levels to the ground states in one or more jumps.

For example, when the electron jumps from all the energy levels higher than n = 1, i.e., n = 2, 3, 4, 5... to n = 1 energy level, the lines obtained fall in the ultraviolet region, these lines are called Lyman series.

Similarly, the lines obtained, when an electron jumps to the second energy level (n = 2) from higher levels (n = 3, 4, 5, 6) fall in the visible region. These are called the Balmer series.

In a similar manner, the transition from higher energy levels to n = 3 series produces the Paschen series. Similarly, Brackett and Pfund series correspond to jumps from higher energy levels to n = 4 and n = 5 energy levels respectively. Thus are summarized below **(Fig. 10.5)**:

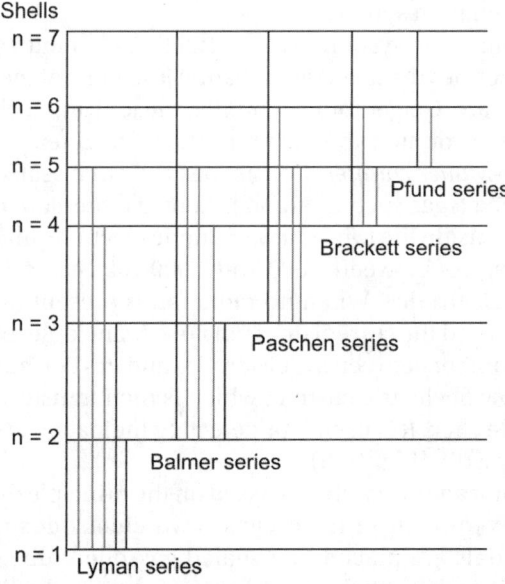

Fig. 10.5: Orbits of an atom.

Lyman series from n = 2, 3, 4, 5... to n = 1
Balmer series from n = 3, 4, 5, 6... to n = 2
Paschen series from n = 4, 5, 6, 7... to n = 3
Brackett series from n = 4, 5, 6, 7... to n = 4
Pfund series from n = 5, 6, 7... to n = 5

Bohr's theory helped in calculating the energy of the electron in a particular orbit of the hydrogen atom and that is:

$$E_n = 2\pi^2 \, me/N^2h^2$$

Weaknesses

- Bohr's model of an atom could not explain the time spectra of atoms containing more than one electron called multi-electron atom.
- Bohr's theory failed to account for the effect of magnetic fields on the spectra of atoms or ions called Zeeman effect.
- Bohr's theory does not provide any clue to explain the shapes of molecules arising out of the directional bonding between atoms.

Applications

Detection of Radioactivity and Monitoring

- To evaluate radiation hazards, periodic readings need to be made in the field around a source or sources of radiation.
- Area monitoring is a term used to describe the periodic or continuous determination of dosage levels in working areas around various radiation sources.
- Each monitoring system uses a detecting element and a device that transcribes the detected radiation into units of measurement. Examples are, Geiger muller counter, the ionization chamber, the scintillation counter, and the proportional counter.
  - *Geiger-Muller counter:* Consist basically of a sealed glass tube in which a gas such as argon is kept at a pressure of above 0.1 atoms, inside the tube is a wire anode electrode and a cathode. A voltage of between 1,000 and 2,000 volts is present between these electrodes. When no radiation is present the gas is not ionized and the current does not flow. A single electron entering the chamber between the electrodes initiates lionization causing the flow of electric current, which is then transformed into an audible click. It is useful for detecting radioactivity in radiation survey work **(Fig. 10.6)**.
  - The ionization chamber is based on the principle that radiation causes ionization in the gas. Two electrodes at opposite potentials are placed in a sealed gas-filled tube. Passage of radiations through the chamber produce ions that are attracted

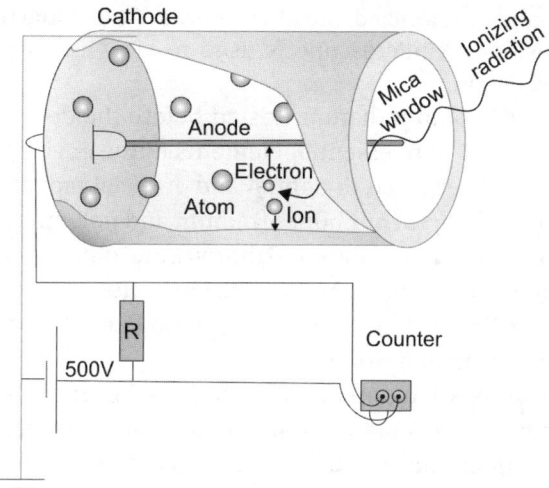

Fig. 10.6: Gigger-Muller counter.

to the oppositely charged electrode. The current produced in this apparatus is read on a meter.

- *The proportional counting chamber.* This differs from the previous apparatus in that, it produces a pulse whose strength is proportional to the energy of the entering ionizing radiations. This apparatus is useful in measuring alpha radiations. It can also distinguish alpha from beta and gamma radiations because of the energy differences between these three kinds of radiations.
- *Scintillation counters:* Contain crystals that liberate light when exposed to radiations. The flashes of light are too faint to be seen and are therefore converted into electrical impulses through the use of a photomultiplier tube. Scintillation counters are useful for rapid counting and for discriminating between different types of radiations that are emitted spontaneously.
  - Some counters are reduced to a pocket-size that can be conveniently carried by persons working in an area where radiations are present.
  - In addition to the counters mentioned, the electroscope is a direct viewing apparatus especially employed for measuring gamma radiations. A useful type is the quartz fiber electroscope. This is sealed in a chamber in which a metalized quartz fiber is mounted so that it is insulated from the inner wall of the chamber. A battery puts an initial charge on the fiber and the fiber is deflected. When the gas in the

chamber is ionized, the fiber returns to the initial uncharged position. A microscope is used to view and measure the deflection.

Radioactivity and radiation existed before the development of life on Earth and were essential elements of the environment. We are continuously exposed to natural and artificial radiations. These radionuclides are part of our bones (radium and polonium), muscles (radiocarbon, radiopotassium, and thoron), and other tissues and are emitting ionizing radiation. Nuclear fusion in the sun is responsible for the radiation which is essential for life on Earth. So we are living in a radioactive natural world.

Radioisotopes have many applications in medicine. One of the most important is radioimmunoassay. This is a technique that detects and quantifies minute amounts of components in tissues such as hormones or enzymes. It compares the component's ability to bind with an antibody or other proteins to determine if it is the same component that has been radioactively tagged in the laboratory.

Radioisotopes could be released from nuclear fuel cycles or naturally occurring radioactive substances (NORM) mining activities, as well as an accidental radioactive material released into the atmosphere. Protective actions must be taken immediately. The main goal is to concentrate on radioisotopes' applications and radiological protection.

■ RADIATION AND RADIOISOTOPES

The basic building block of matter is the atom proposed by John in the atomic theory. As we know the atom is composed of a positively charged nucleus, surrounded by a number of negatively charged electrons and so the whole atom is electrically neutral. The number of protons and neutrons present in the nucleus, called atomic number (Z), is known as mass number (A). An element›s atomic number is the same. However, elements with different mass numbers are called "isotopes". An unstable nucleus will result if the nucleus has either too many protons or neutrons. An unstable nucleus will vibrate continuously and attempt to stabilize itself by radioactive decay. The number of neutrons in a nucleus determines whether it is radioactive or not. Radioisotopes are radioactive elements. They can be produced naturally or artificially by accelerators and nuclear reactors. Rutherford and Soddy discovered that radioactivity was directly linked to the state of the atomic nucleus.

Radioactivity and nuclear reactions can happen at the time of emitting radiation from unstable nuclei. Radioactivity is the spontaneous disintegration of a nucleus to produce different types of nuclei or a lower energy nucleus. This results in the emission of alpha (α), beta (β), and gamma (γ) radiation and known as radioactivity. Henry Becquerel discovered radioactivity in 1896. Rutherford discovered alpha, beta, and their ionizing properties in 1899. Villard discovered gamma in 1900. The nucleus reacts with another particle or nucleus to produce nuclear reactions that result in the emission of radiation. Sometimes, the final product can also be radioactive. These radiations can be either electromagnetic (X-rays or γ-rays), or particle-like α and β. Rutherford discovered the nuclear reactions in 1917.

Radiation Classification

Radiation is divided into two main types based on its ability to ionize matter, ionizing radiation and non-ionizing radiation.

Ionizing Radiation

Radiation that passes through matter and breaks down the bonds between atoms or molecules and removes an electron, is known as ionization radiation. It can pass through living organisms or matter and produce a variety of effects. Radioactive decay, nuclear fission, and fusion are the main sources of ionizing radiation. Particle accelerators and extremely hot objects also produce it. There are two types of ionizing radiation: direct and indirect.

Direct Ionizing Radiation

Directly ionizing radiation deposits heat in the medium by direct Coulomb interaction of the ionizing charged particle and orbital electrons. This can be done to atoms by α, β, protons and heavy ions.

Ionizing radiations such as alpha (α), beta (β), and gamma (γ) except neutron, are created from unstable nuclei in an atom that is undergoing radioactive decay.

Alpha Radiation

There are some naturally occurring heavy nuclei that have an atomic number between 82 to 92 decay by alpha emission, in which the parent nucleus loses mass by 4 units and charges by 2 units and becomes a new atom. An α-particle is a helium nucleus ($_2He^4$) consisting of 2 protons and 2 neutrons. They are positively charged moving with a speed of about 2×10^7 ms^{-1} ionizing the surrounding gas and photographic plate. They can cause fluorescence in ZnS.

The parent nucleus ($_ZX^A$) is transformed by the following equation:

$_ZX^A = {}_{Z-2}X^{A-4} + {}_2He^{4+} + Q$ (energy)

$_{92}U^{238} = {}_{90}Th^{234} + {}_2He^{4+} + Q$ (energy)

Uranium thorium alpha particle.

Beta radiation

These are either fast electrons or positrons. They are formed from weak interaction decay of a proton or neutron in nuclei that contain excess of this nucleon. A neutron-rich nucleus can be transformed into a proton through the emission of beta particles or antineutrino. It can also be transformed into a neutron in nuclei containing rich protons by releasing neutrino or positron. Beta particles are negatively charged moving with speed of 2.97×10^8 ms^{-1}. These radiations have a high penetrating power but less ionizing power than alpha particles. ˇ They can also cause fluorescence in ZnS as alpha particles.

The parent nucleus ($_ZX^A$) is transformed by the following equation:

$_ZX^A = {}_{Z+1}X^A + {}_{-1}\beta^0 + Q$ (energy) [n = p + 0 β^- + ν]

$_{90}Th^{234} = {}_{91}Pa^{234} + {}_{-1}\beta^0$

Thorium protactinium beta particle

Indirect Ionizing Radiation

Indirectly ionizing radiation deposits heat in the medium in two steps. The first step sees charged particles being released into the medium. The second step is where the charged particles are released into the medium and deposit energy through direct Coulomb interaction. This can be done with atoms such as photons, electrons, X-rays, gamma rays, and neutrons.

Gamma Radiation

Gamma radiation is the most common form of nuclear excitation and can also occur due to internal conversion. They are electromagnetic rays like light and traveling with the speed of light 3×10^8 ms^{-1} have the highest penetrating powers, electrically neutral and least ionizing powers.

X-ray Radiation

The electron cloud around the nucleus produces X-rays. Roentgen discovered them in 1895. X-rays can be produced in X-ray tubes by fast-moving electrons that are suddenly stopped by the target.

Neutron Radiation

It is a neutral particle and causes ionization indirectly through the emission of gamma rays and charged particles while interacting with matter. These charged particles cause ionization. It is more powerful than gamma radiation and can be stopped with thin concrete or paraffin barriers. They can be produced by nuclear reactions and spontaneous fission within nuclear reactors.

Nonionizing Radiation

Nonionizing radiation refers to electromagnetic radiation that does not produce ionization. It has enough energy to excite, but not to create ions in matter. Nonionizing radiations include radio waves, microwaves, and ultraviolets. While nonionizing radiation is vital for life, excessive exposure can cause adverse biological effects.

Natural and Artificial Radiation Sources

Two important sources of radiation are man-made and natural.

Natural background radiation is the radiation that surrounds us. Every living organism, including man, has been exposed to ionizing radiations from various sources, they come from cosmic rays, primordial radionuclides, such as ^{232}Th, ^{235}U, and ^{238}U, as well as their decay products, as well as single-occurring radionuclides ^{40}K and ^{87}Rb that are found in the earth's crust, soil, rocks, and other materials. Natural radiation originates from three main sources: terrestrial, extraterrestrial, and internal sources (intake of radionuclides or their daughter products).

Terrestrial Radiation Sources

Terra is the Latin word for earth. The radiation that originated from the crust of the earth is known as terrestrial radiation. The sources of terrestrial radiation are the primordial radionuclides (^{238}U and ^{232}Th), which are found in different amounts in soil, rocks, and water. The majority of natural radiation comes from ^{40}K, ^{238}U, and ^{232}Th and their decay products. They undergo radioactive decay series before becoming stable isotopes. These radioactive series are naturally occurring radioactive series that have been around since the formation of the earth. Each series nuclei decay by emitting alpha, beta, and gamma particles to become stable (lead). These radioisotopes, which are chemically bound with minerals in soils and rocks, pose no biological dangers other than radon and thoron. The noble radioactive gas noble radon (a product of uranium decay series) and thoron (a product of thorium decay series) can be inhaled to cause lung cancer. UNSCEAR and WHO report that radon and its progeny are second-leading causes of lung cancer, after smoking tobacco.

^{40}K is easily absorbed by the body through drinking water, eating foods, and breathing air. ^{40}K is absorbed quickly through the stomach tract and into the bloodstream. The ^{40}K rapidly enters the bloodstream, where it is distributed to all tissues and organs, mainly muscles. This isotope delivers approximately 18 millirems (mrem), to the soft tissues and 14 mrem, to the bones each year. ^{40}K may pose both internal and external health risks.

Extraterrestrial Radiations

Extraterrestrial radiations (or cosmic radiations) are high-energy radiations or subatomic particles that originate mainly from stars that come from space and bombard the earth and all living creatures. The cosmic ray radiation is composed of about 85% protons, and 14% of alpha particles (helium ions), that hit the earth's atmosphere and consist of a mixture of charged particles like electrons, and protons, and alpha-particles. There is also a small amount of heavier nuclei. These radiations are extremely energetic and can range from 10^2 MeV to more than 10^{14} MeV. The interaction of cosmic charged particles with the earth's magnetic field and atmosphere results in the formation of the cosmic ray shower, which is typically beta or gamma radiation. Due to variations in elevation and the effects of the earth's magnetic field, the dose of cosmic radiation can vary in different areas of the globe. The upper troposphere is where the cosmic radiations are stronger. The cosmic radiation dose rises with altitude. During flights, crew members receive an additional dose of around 2.2 mSv y^{-1}. The annual cosmic radiation doses around the globe are therefore estimated to be between 0.26 and 2.01 mSv y.

The cosmic radiation interacts directly with the molecules and atoms in the atmosphere. This results in a series of secondary radioisotopes in the form of protons, neutrons, and charged/uncharged particles of different energies. These radioisotopes include ^{3}H, ^{7}Be, and ^{14}C. These cosmogonic radionuclides eventually reach the earth's surface, where they can be incorporated into living organisms. They also contribute to natural radiation exposures. The annual equivalent dose of cosmogonic radionuclides to the earth's surface is 12 mSv (14C), 0.15 mSv (22Na), 0.01 mSv (^{3}H), and 0.03 mSv (^{7}Be). The most significant is ^{14}C.

Internal Sources of Radiation

Radioactive material can enter the body through eating, drinking, and injections (from certain medical procedures, radon/thoron, and their progeny). If inhaled or injected in large quantities, the radioactive material can pose a serious health risk.

Artificial or Manmade Radiation

Human beings are also exposed to radiation from nuclear installations, nuclear explosions, nuclear fuel cycle, radioactive waste releases from nuclear reactor operations, and other industrial, and medical such as diagnostic X-rays, nuclear therapy, and agricultural uses of radioisotopes. It can also be generated by consumer products like TVs, luminous watches, dials, and radioactive materials (gas and coal). This includes the whole sequence of mining, milling, and actual production of nuclear power plants, as well as the residual fallout from nuclear weapons testing and accidents.

Radioisotope Applications

Radioisotopes play a major role in improving human life quality. There are some international organizations such as the International Atomic Energy Agency and International Commission on Radiation Protection to identify the needs and provide the infrastructure to support nuclear technology.

Radiotracer

The first report of the clinical use of radioisotopes occurred in 1937 when radio phosphorus was administered to the patient. Since that time there has been phenomenal growth in the use of radioisotopes for diagnosis and treatment.

Radiotracers are used extensively in medicine, agriculture, and industry as well as in fundamental research. A Radiotracer can be described as a radioactive element or compound that is added to a nonradioactive element to examine the dynamic behavior and chemical, biological, and physical changes in a system. It emits traceable radiation back. There are over 160 radioisotopes used in various fields. Some of the radioisotopes and their applications are presented in the following **Table 10.1:**

Table 10.1		
Radioisotope	*Half-life*	*Applications*
Bismuth-213	45.59 minutes	It is an alpha emitter used in cancer treatment, such as targeted alpha therapy (TAT).
Cesium-131	9.7 days	It emits photon radiation within the X-ray spectrum used in the brachytherapy treatment of malignant tumors.
Chromium-51	28 days	Useful in the diagnosis of gastrointestinal bleeding and labeling platelets.

Contd...

Contd...

Radioisotope	Half-life	Applications
Cobalt-60	5.27 years	This is used to control the growth of cancerous cells.
Iodine-131	8 days	Widely used for treating thyroid cancer, diagnosing and imaging the thyroid and renal blood flow.
Iron-59	46 days	Used in iron metabolism studies in the spleen.
Lead-212	10.6 h	Use in TAT for cancers.
Palladium-103	17 days	This is used to create brachytherapy permanent implant seeds for early-stage prostate carcinoma. Soft X-rays.
Potassium-42	12.36 h	Used to study the distribution of potassium in bodily fluids, and to locate brain tumours.
Radium-223	11.4 Days	This is used to treat prostate cancers that have spread to the bones.
Rhenium-186	3.71 days	This is used to treat bone cancer pain and also for imaging purposes.
Sodium-24	15 h	This is used to study electrolytes in the body.
Ytterbium-169	32 days	Useful for cerebrospinal fluid studies in the brain.
Cobalt-57	272 days	It is used to determine the size of an organ and in vitro diagnostic kits.
Copper-64	13 h	This is used for PET imaging of tumors, and also for cancer therapy.
Fluorine-18	110 minutes	Useful as fluorothymidine FLT.
Gallium-67	78 h	This is used to locate inflammatory lesions and tumors (infections).
Indium-111	2.8 Days	Brain studies, colon transit, and infection.
Iodine-123	13 h	This is used to diagnose thyroid function.
Rubidium-82	1.26 minutes	Convenient PET agent for myocardial perfusion imaging.
Thallium-201	73 h	This is used to locate low-grade lymphomas.

Radiotracer is an essential and advanced diagnostic tool for radiotherapy and medicine.

Diagnostic Purpose

Technetium (^{99}Tc) is the most commonly used radioactivity isotope in the radioactive tracer. To locate brain tumors, inject intravenously ^{99}Tc into the head and scan the head using suitable scanners.

To study the function of malfunctioning thyroid glands, ^{131}I, ^{132}I, and ^{123}I were recently used. Compounds containing ^{131}I are also used to study kidney function. ^{33}P can be used for DNA sequencing. Tritium (3H) has been used in biochemical research as a tracer. ^{14}C is used extensively to track the progression of organic molecules through metabolic pathways.

The most recent advancement is positron emission tomography (PET), which allows for more accurate and precise detection of tumors within the body. A positron-emitting radionuclide (e.g., ^{13}N, ^{15}O, ^{18}F, etc.). It is administered to the patient and accumulates in the target tissues. It emits a positron, which quickly combines with nearby electrons. This causes simultaneous emission of two different g-rays. A PET camera detects these g-rays and gives precise information about their origin. This technique can also be used for brain and cardiac imaging.

Complementary X-ray tomography (CT scans). A radioactive tracer emits gamma radiation or single photons, which a gamma camera can detect. A computer can use these emissions to create an image. CT scans target specific areas of the body like the neck and chest or an organ like the thyroid.

Therapeutic

The most popular therapeutic use for radioisotopes in cancer treatment is ^{60}Co. Sometimes, wires and sealed needles containing radioactive Isotopes such as ^{192}Ir and ^{125}I can be directly inserted into cancerous tissue. As long as the needle/wire remains in place, the radiations from radioisotopes target the tumor. These are then removed after the treatment is completed. This is a common treatment for mouth, breast, lung, and uterine cancers. ^{131}I can be used to treat thyroid cancers and other abnormalities. ^{32}P can be used to treat excess red blood cells in the bone marrow.

For total sterilization of the diets of immunocompromised patients, astronauts, military personnel, adventure sports, and military personnel, higher doses of radiation can be used.

Agricultural Research

Research in agricultural science is focusing on the development of high-yielding plants, oilseeds and other economically valuable crops, as well as the protection of the plant from insects. In order to increase crop variety and improve mutation breeding, irradiated wheat, rice, maize, and cotton seeds are going through profound genetic changes. These crops have higher yields and are more resistant to disease.

The sterile insect technique (SIT) is the best method for controlling pests and insects. To sterilize insects that have been raised in large numbers, radiation is used. This allows them to not produce offspring, but they can still be sexually competitive. It enhances crop production and preserves natural resources with biodiversity.

Food Preservation and Sterilization

According to the WHO, 25–35% of world food production is susceptible to pests, bugs, bacteria, and fungi, causing great economic losses for the country. Irradiating food has many more benefits than traditional methods. Food irradiation is not recommended by all radiations. Only three types of radiation are recommended including ^{60}Co, ^{137}Cs and X-rays. Food products are subject to intense controlled radiation to kill pests, bugs, and parasites. This not only extends shelf life but also decreases nutrition by degrading vitamins A, B_1 (thiamin), and C.

Radiated potatoes can be kept at a higher temperature, around 15° Celsius by inhibition of bulbs or tubers. This will not only save energy but also prevent sweetening from potatoes that is often caused by low temperatures.

These fruits, all types of mangoes, can be irradiated at the hard mature pre-climacteric phase at 0.25–0.75 kGy to delay the ripening process for about 7 days. This will improve shelf-life up to 30 days, at 12–14°C in modified environments.

Poor handling and processing conditions can lead to spices becoming contaminated with microbial pathogens and insect eggs while being transported. Semi-processed and processed foods can be contaminated with microbes and pathogens. This can lead to spoilage and pose a risk to consumers. A 10 kGy dose will result in near sterility, or commercial sterility, while still retaining the natural properties of spices.

Industrial Use

Industry uses radioisotopes to check for blocked pipes and detect oil leakage. A small amount of radioactive ^{24}Na can be placed in an enclosed ball that is allowed to move through pipes with water. A detector is used to monitor the radioisotope-containing moving ball. The obstruction is indicated if the ball's movement stops.

Radioisotope ^{24}Na mixed with oil in underground pipes is another example. Radioisotopes can also be used to monitor fluid flow, and filtration, detect leaks, and gauge engine wear.

Industries need to monitor their production processes in order to ensure quality and control. Quality control devices that use the unique radiation properties of radiation are used to monitor production. These devices are known as nuclear gauges. They are more useful at extreme temperatures, in harmful chemical processes, molten glass, and metals. They are used to measure thicknesses of sheet materials such as metals, textiles, and paper, and to inspect the integrity of welds and metal parts across many industries..

Radioisotope Exposure Effects

Radiation that passes through the material causes the bonds to break down by removing an electron from one or more atoms or molecules. This can cause physical, chemical and biological changes. Ionizing radiation concentrates large amounts of energy in highly concentrated areas of irradiated material. This energy can cause damage by interaction with nuclei and orbiting electrons. This energy interaction can alter the material structure, causing changes in the mechanical properties of bulk materials. Radiation-induced degradation technology (RIDA) is a novel application for developing viscose and pulp, paper, pharmaceutical production, food preservation, and natural bioactive agents industries.

Radiation Effects on the Body

Health effects refer to the harmful effects of radiation exposure on human health. A trail of ionized molecules and atoms are the result of all physical interactions between incident radiation and cells. Radiation interacts directly with the DNA of sensitive sites in the tissue to cause damage through breaking chemical bonds. Interaction of primary radiation with the DNA of the tissue produces chemically active free radicals through ionization. The figure below shows both direct and indirect damage to DNA caused by radiation.

It is caused by the chemical radicals that are generated by radiation and interact with water molecules. Indirect action accounts for about 80% tissue. Because they can travel far enough to cause chemical changes in critical areas of biological structures, free radicals are crucial. Free radicals can cause chemical damage by destroying DNA.

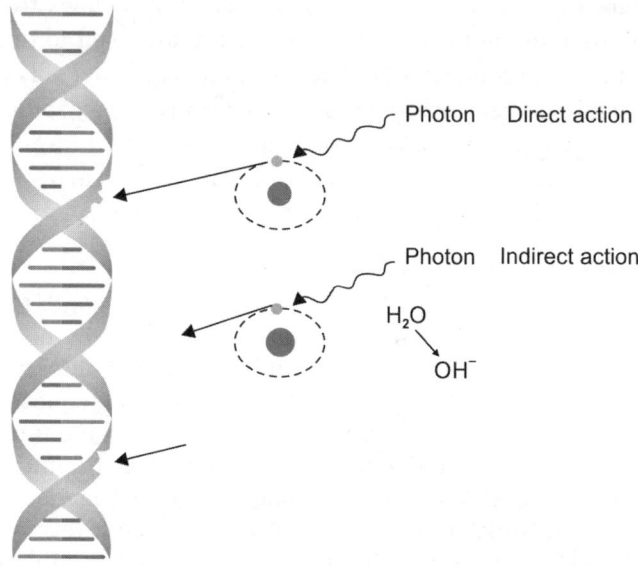

DNA is a double-helix structure. If radiation/free radicals only break one strand, the damage can be easily repaired using the opposite strand as a template. Double strand breakage makes it impossible to repair the cell. This can lead to mutations, or changes in the DNA code that cause cell death or cancer. These molecules can be repaired by natural biological processes to a certain degree, but this depends on the severity of the damage.

Radiation damage can have long-term or short-term effects. Acute radiation effects are those that result from prolonged exposure to radiation for a short time. A chronic effect, or delayed effect, is a small amount of radiation that has been exposed for a longer time. If the dose is greater than 500 mSv, then deterministic effects can be severe. The severity of effects are shown in **Table 10.2:**

Table 10.2

Effective dose	Time of exposure	Effects
<1 Sv	Weeks Very short period	Reduction of white blood cells Recovery is good
About 2 Sv	1 h within one week 3-4 weeks	Nausea, headache, or vomiting 50% decreases in lymphocytes, 50% decreases in thrombocyte levels It is possible to recover quickly
3 Sv	From hours to days After few days Within one week or more	Radiation sickness can cause nausea, vomiting, and fatigue as well as loss of appetite, infection, infections, dehydration, and hair loss. The patient may feel better Recovering well
4 Sv	Few weeks	Intestine mucous membrane and bone marrow tissue have been damaged
5–6 Sv	—	There is a strong chance of death
>6 Sv	—	It is unlikely that you will survive for more than a few weeks.
>10 Sv	Within 2 weeks	Death will result from the irreparable damage to the mucous membranes of the intestines.
50 Sv	Within hours Within one day	Loss of consciousness and damage to the central nervous system could result in death.

The delay in the time between exposure and the observed health effects is due to chronic exposure. These health effects can include cancer, as well as other outcomes like cataracts and benign tumors.

To minimize radiation exposure for medical professionals, it is possible to follow as low as reasonably practicable (ALARA) or to use personnel shielding options (e.g. two-piece wraparound aprons and thyroid shields) to reduce scattered X-ray levels. Dose limits are not applicable to patients who are exposed for medical reasons. Medical radiation is not subject to dose limits. Instead, doctors use the diagnostic reference level (DRL), which is a reference value for medical radiation.

Radiation exposure risk must be reduced by minimizing medical radiation exposure. Furthermore, ionizing radiation-related examinations must be optimized to reduce radiation exposure. Justification refers to the medically justified and clinically useful examination. Optimization refers to the use of doses as low as possible in order to achieve the diagnostic task.

Public exposure control is usually achieved by controlling radiation at the source, rather than in the surrounding environment. The ICRP recommends that the dose limits not exceed 1 mSv y^{-1} (excluding normal background radiation). In exceptional circumstances, however, a higher dose limit can be permitted for a single year, provided that the average of 5 years does not exceed 1 mSv y^{-1}.

The following parameters can be used to control occupational exposure:

Distance: To reduce radiation exposure, the distance between the source worker and the worker should be great.

Time: Radiation dose is directly proportional to the amount of radiation received. The radiation dose should therefore be kept as short as possible.

Shielding: Different materials can be used depending on the type of radiation. High-atomic numbered elements for gamma radiation are used because the rate at which energy is lost is directly proportional Z^5. High absorption cross-sections and low-atomic number elements are used to shield neutrons. Hydrogen and hydrogen-based materials work well for neutron shielding. We can use plastic to create a barrier that protects against high-energy beta radiation.

■ RADIATION PROTECTION LIMITS

The normal exposure of individuals resulting from all relevant practices should be subject to dose limits to ensure that no individual is exposed to a risk that is judged to be unacceptable.

The Nuclear Regulatory Commission (NRC) and the Environmental Protection Agency (EPA) have established three layers of radiation protection limits to protect the public against potential health risks from exposure to radioactive liquid discharges (effluents) from nuclear power plant operations.

CHAPTER 10: Nuclear Physics

Table 10.3: Dose limitations.

Part of the body	Occupational exposure	Public exposure
Whole body (Effective dose)	20 mSv/year averaged over 5 consecutive years; 30 mSv in any single year	1 mSv/y
Lens of eyes (Equivalent dose)	150 mSv in a year	15 mSv/y
Skin (Equivalent dose)	500 mSv in a year	50 mSv/y
Extremities (Hands and feet) Equivalent dose	500 mSv in a year	-

For pregnant radiation workers, after the declaration of pregnancy 1 mSv on the embryo/fetus should not exceed.

Layer 1:3 mrem per year ALARA (As Low as in Reasonably Achievable) Objective- Appendix 1 to 10 CFR Part 50

The NRC requires that nuclear plant operators must keep radiation doses from gas and liquid effluents as low as reasonably achievable (ALARA) to people offsite. For liquid effluent releases, such as diluted tritium, the ALARA annual offsite dose objective is 3 mrem to the whole body and 10 mrem to any organ of a maximally exposed individual who lives in close proximity to the plant boundary. This ALARA objective is 3% of the annual public dose limit of 100 mrem.

The NRC selected the 3 mrem and 10 mrem per year values because they are a fraction of the natural background radiation dose, a fraction of the annual public dose limit, and an attainable objective that nuclear power plants could meet. Power plants that meet these objectives are considered to be ALARA in reducing exposures to the general public from nuclear power plant effluents.

Nuclear power plant operators must monitor the authorized releases (effluents) from their plants. If a given nuclear power plant exceeds half of these radiation dose levels in a calendar quarter, the plant operator is required to investigate the cause, initiate appropriate corrective actions, and report the actions to the NRC within 30 days from the end of the quarter.

Layer 2:25 mrem per year standard—10 CFR 20.1301 (e)

In 1979, EPA developed a radiation dose standard of 25 mrem to the whole body, 75 mrem to the thyroid, 25 mrem to any other organ of an individual member of the public. The NRC incorporated these EPA standards into its regulation in 1981, and all nuclear power plants must now meet these requirements. These standards are specific to facilities that are involved in generating nuclear power (commonly called the 'uranium fuel cycle'), including where nuclear fuel is milled, manufactured, and used in nuclear power reactors. EPA determines the basis of the standards by comparing the cost-effectiveness of various dose limits in reducing potential health risks from operations of these types of facilities. EPA assumes the standards would be able to meet for up to four fuel cycle facilities at one location. Notably, the NRC's ALARA objectives are lower than these EPA standards.

Layer 3: 100 mrem per year limit—10 CFR 20.1301 (a) (1)

The NRC's final layer of protection of public health and safety is a dose limit of 100 mrem per year for individual members of the public. This limit applies to everyone, including academics, universities, and medical facilities that use radioactive material.

The NRC adopted the 100 mrem per year dose limit from the 1990 recommendations of the International Commission on Radiological Protection (ICRP). The ICRP is an organization of international radiation scientists who provide recommendations regarding radiation protection-related activities, including dose limits. The basis of the ICRP recommendation of 100 mrem per year is that a lifetime of exposure at this limit would result in very small health risk and is roughly equivalent to background radiation from natural sources.

Basic Three Factors for Radiation Protection (Working Personnel and Public)

Time
- Exposure to radiation source is directly proportional to the time
- Reduce the period of exposure to radiation to reduce the dose received from the source.

Distance
- Increase distance from source to decrease exposure rate.
- $I_1 d_1^2 = I_2 d_2^2$ (Inverse-square law)
- Double the distance from the source; dose-rate falls to ¼ the original value.
- Halve the distance from the source; the dose-rate increases to 4 times the original value.

❖ More the distance from the source—The lesser the radiation

Shielding
❖ Use an appropriate shielding material or protection devices
❖ Shielding reduces exposure rate
❖ Use large shielding thickness (High-Z materials e.g., Lead, Steel, Concrete, etc.)—to reduce the exposure rate of gamma/X-ray radiation.

■ INSTRUMENTS USED FOR DETECTION OF IONIZING RADIATION, X-RAYS

Ionizing radiation, such as X-rays, alpha rays, beta rays, and gamma rays, remains undetectable by the senses, and the damage it causes to the body is cumulative, related to the total dose received. Therefore, workers who are exposed to radiation, such as radiographers, nuclear power plant workers, doctors using radiotherapy, workers in laboratories using radionuclides, and some HAZMAT teams are required to wear instruments that can keep a record of their exposure, to verify that it is below legally prescribed limits. Ionizing radiations can be measured or monitored by Dosimeters, Geiger counters, and scintillation counters.

❖ **Dosimeters:** Dosimeters measure an absolute dose received over a period of time. Ion-chamber dosimeters resemble pens and can be clipped to one's clothing. Common types of wearable dosimeters for ionizing radiation include:
- Quartz fiber dosimeter
- Film badge dosimeter
- Thermoluminescent dosimeter
- Solid-state (MOSFET or silicon diode) dosimeter
    ◆ Film-badge dosimeters enclose a piece of photographic film, which will become exposed as the radiation passes through it. Ion-chamber dosimeters must be periodically recharged, and the result logged. Film-badge dosimeters must be developed as photographic emulsions so the exposures can be counted and logged; once developed, they are discarded. Another type of dosimeter is the TLD (Thermoluminescent Dosimeter). These dosimeters contain crystals that emit visible light when heated, in direct proportion to their total radiation exposure. Like ion-chamber dosimeters, TLDs can be re-used after they have been 'read.' Common types of wearable dosimeters for ionizing radiation includes.

- **Geiger counters:** Geiger counters are used to detect ionizing radiation (usually beta particles and gamma rays, but certain models can detect alpha particles). An inert gas-filled tube (usually helium, neon, or argon with halogens added) briefly conducts electricity when a particle or photon of radiation makes the gas conductive. The tube amplifies this conduction by a cascade effect and outputs a current pulse, which is then often displayed by a needle or lamp and/or audible clicks. Modern instruments can report radioactivity over several orders of magnitude.
- **Scintillation counters:** A scintillation counter measures ionizing radiation. The sensor, called a scintillator, consists of a transparent crystal, usually phosphor, plastic (usually containing anthracene), or organic liquid (see liquid scintillation counting) that fluoresces when struck by ionizing radiation. A sensitive photomultiplier tube (PMT) measures the light from the crystal. The PMT is attached to an electronic amplifier and other electronic equipment to count and possibly quantify the amplitude of the signals produced by the photomultiplier.

■ QUESTIONS

Q.1: Radioiodine is given to patients with hyperthyroidism. Explain.

Q.2: Which measures are taken to reduce exposure to radioactivity in hospitals?

Q.3: Use of radioisotopes in cancer therapy. Discuss.

Q.4: Use of film badges by radiographers. Explain.

■ BIBLIOGRAPHY

1. Beyer HF, Shevelko VP. Introduction to the Physics of Highly Charged Ions. CRC Press, 2003.
2. Choppin, Gregory R. Liljenzin Jan-Olov Rydberg Jan. Radiochemistry and Nuclear Chemistry. Elsevier, 2001.
3. Demtröder W. Atoms, Molecules and Photons: An Introduction to Atomic, Molecular- and Quantum Physics (1st edition). Springer, 2002.
4. Fowles GR. Introduction to Modern Optics. Courier Dover Publications, 1989.
5. Gangopadhyaya M. Indian Atomism: History and Sources. Atlantic Highlands, New Jersey: Humanities Press, 1981.
6. Goodstein DL. States of Matter. Courier Dover Publications, 2002.
7. Harrison ER. Masks of the Universe: Changing Ideas on the Nature of the Cosmos. Cambridge University Press, 2003.
8. Jevremovic T. Nuclear Principles in Engineering. Springer, 2005.
9. Knoll G. Radiation Detection and Measurement. John Wiley and Sons, 1999.

10. L'Annunziata MF. Handbook of Radioactivity Analysis. Academic Press, 2003.
11. Lequeux J. The Interstellar Medium. Springer, 2005.
12. Levere TH. Transforming Matter: A History of Chemistry from Alchemy to the Buckyball. The Johns Hopkins University Press, 2001.
13. MacGregor MH. The Enigmatic Electron. Oxford University Press, 1992.
14. Manuel O. Origin of Elements in the Solar System: Implications of Post-1957 Observations. Springer, 2001.
15. Mazo RM. Brownian Motion: Fluctuations, Dynamics, and Applications. Oxford University Press, 2002.
16. Moran BT. Distilling Knowledge: Alchemy, Chemistry, and the Scientific Revolution, 2005.
17. Myers R. The Basics of Chemistry. Greenwood Press, 2003.
18. Padilla MJ, Miaoulis I, Cyr M. Prentice Hall Science Explorer: Chemical Building Blocks. Upper Saddle River, New Jersey USA: Prentice-Hall, Inc., 2002.
19. Pfeffer JI, Nir S. Modern Physics: An Introductory Text. Imperial College Press, 2000.
20. Scerri ER. The Periodic Table. Oxford University Press, 2007.
21. Shultis JK, Faw RE. Fundamentals of Nuclear Science and Engineering. CRC Press, 2002.
22. Siegfried R. From Elements to Atoms: A History of Chemical Composition. DIANE, 2002.
23. Woan G. The Cambridge Handbook of Physics. Cambridge University Press, 2000.
24. Zaider M, Rossi HH. Radiation Science for Physicians and Public Health Workers. Springer, 2001.
25. Radiological Protection Principles. Available from https://www.aerb.gov.in/english/radiation-protection-principle. Cited 29-05-2022

CHAPTER 11

Electronics in Nursing

Suresh K Sharma, Rakhi Gaur

CHAPTER OUTLINE
- Principles of Electronics
- Capacitors
- Transistors
- Transducers
- Common Electric Equipment Used in Patient Care

■ INTRODUCTION

The use of electronics can be observed in most of the basic and advanced healthcare practices. Advancement in science in technology has brought the boom in the use of electronics in healthcare practices. One can observe the use of electronic thermometers for recording patient's temperature, and electronic blood pressure monitoring devices. Patient bedside automatic monitors can automatically detect the vital signs, ECG, oxygen saturation, carbon-dioxide saturation, apnea status of patients, etc. These monitors are frequently observed in intensive care units (ICU) and operation theatres (OT). Recently, the use of advanced ventilators and robots in healthcare practices are new examples of the use of electronics in nursing.

Electronics is that branch of physics and technology that deals with the electrical circuits involving active components such as diodes, transistors, etc. Active components of an electrical circuit control the electron flow and are able to amplify weak signals, e.g. battery, transistor, etc. Most electronic devices use semiconductor components to control electron flow. Before semiconductor and solid-state devices, vacuum tubes were the prime electronic components. Electronic circuits can be divided into two categories:

- ❖ **Analog Circuits:** Analog circuits use continuous voltages. They perform amplification, etc. on continuous signals.

- ❖ **Digital Circuits:** Digital circuits are those electronic circuits that work on a number of discrete voltage levels. They are the basis of digital calculators, computers, and all modern electronic instruments.
  - *Diode:* A diode is a two-terminal electronic device, made of semiconductor materials, which have a non-linear resistance. Its prominent feature of it is to allow an electric current in one direction while blocking an electric current in opposite direction.
    - ◆ Diodes are the basic building blocks of all electronic circuits. Today, most the diodes are made of silicon or otherwise germanium.

■ PRINCIPLES OF ELECTRONICS

Principles of electronics can be understood by the explanation of the following aspects of electronics.

Vacuum Tubes

In 1883, Thomson Edison an American inventor, noticed in working with his early incandescent lamps that a small current would pass between the hot filament of the lamp and an additional electrode sealed inside the tube when the additional electrode was made positive. The phenomenon did not occur when the electrode was made negative. This was due to the escape of electrons from the surface of the metal. The escape of electrons from the surface of hot metal is known as thermal electron emission or thermionic emission.

Phenomenon

In the tube, this thermionic emission will result in a cluster of electrons around the emitting hot metal and makes the escape of other electrons difficult. By placing a valve in the form of a positive charge plate in the tube, the negatively charged electrons move toward the positive plate, making room for additional electrons to escape from the hot filament. This action results in a flow of electrons or an electric current. If the tube is evacuated of air, the electrons will flow more rapidly from the emitting filament to the positively charged plate.

Types of Vacuum Tubes

- ❖ **Diode tube:** The simplest type of vacuum tube is known as a diode because it contains two electrodes. It consisted of a hot filament at one end of the tube from which electrons "boil off" by thermionic emission into the tube. At the other end of the tube is a metal plate that is charged positively. Because the metal plate is positively

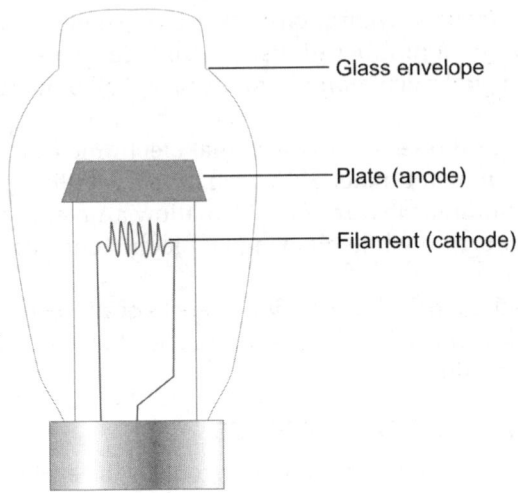

Fig. 11.1: Diode tube.

charged, the electrons that are negatively charged pass from the filament to the plate. The plate can also be negatively charged. When the plate is negatively charged there is no flow of electrons. A third element can be added to the diode tube to make it into a triode tube **(Fig. 11.1)**.

- **Triode tube:** An American inventor Lee de Forest developed the triode tube by introducing a third electrode called the grid to the diode tube is usually made of a mesh screen and is placed between the other two electrodes that is between the cathode and the plate. The grid acts as a control and modifier of the flow of electrons in the vacuum tube **(Fig. 11.2)**.
  - When the grid is made positive, it speeds the movement of the negatively charged electrons through it on their path towards the positive metal tube. When the grid is negatively charged, it slows the speed of the electrons towards the positively charged metal plate. In this way, the grid acts as a regulator and small changes in the electric charge of the grid produce great changes in the flow of electrons through the tube. Because of this structure, the triode tube can be used to amplify a very small current.
- **Multi-element tube:** In addition to diode and triode tube, multi-element tubes have been developed. The simplest of these is the tetrad tube which is another element called a screen is inserted between plates and grid.
- **Pentode tube:** Adding still another element, a suppressor grid between plate and screen produces a pentode tube.

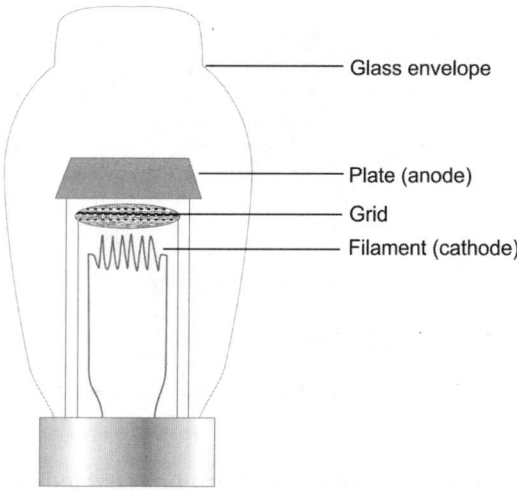

Fig. 11.2: Triode tube.

Uses

A vacuum tube may be used to produce electrical oscillations to "magnify" weak oscillations millions of times or to control oscillations. Electronic computers, radar, and patient monitoring systems are important applications of the vacuum tube.

■ CAPACITORS

A capacitor is a device that stores electrical energy in an electric field. It is a passive electronic component with two terminals. Or a combination of two conductors placed near each other is called a capacitor. These two conductors can be of any shape, e.g. circular, rectangular plates or cylindrical, but generally two parallel conducting rectangular plates are used. These plates are separated by a thin sheet of insulating material called the dielectric. A capacitor is used in a variety of electronic devices to produce even voltages. Its prime objective is to store charges.

A simple example of such a storage device is the parallel-plate capacitor. If positive charges with total charge +Q are deposited on one of the conductors and an equal amount of negative charge –Q is deposited on the second conductor, the capacitor is said to have a charge Q **(Fig. 11.3)**

Working

There is no direct flow of current through the capacitor because of the insulation between the two parallel conducting plates.

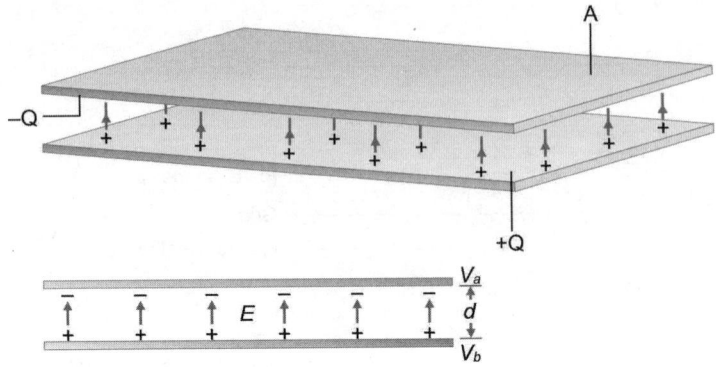

Fig. 11.3: Capacitor.

When placed in a circuit, one plate becomes charged positively and the other negatively. The charge on the positive plate is called the charge on the capacitor and the potential difference between plates is called the potential of the capacitor.

For a given capacitor, the charge Q on the capacitor is proportional to the potential difference V between the plates, i.e.,

$$Q \alpha V$$
$$Q = CV$$

The proportionality constant 'C' is the capacitance of the capacitor. It depends on the shape, size, and distance between the plates of the capacitor and the medium between them. Its SI unit is Farad.

Capacitors store charges, and when a certain force is reached they pass across the insulator, neutralize each other and break the circuit. After this event, charges rebuild on the plates, and the process repeats **(Fig. 11.4)**.

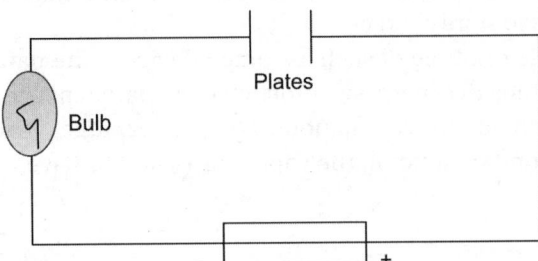

Fig. 11.4: Diagrammatic presentation of a capacitor.

Diagrammatic Presentation

- ❖ These are the two plates of a capacitor.
- ❖ The plate on the capacitor that attaches to the negative terminal of the battery accepts electrons that the battery is producing.
- ❖ The plate on the capacitor that attaches to the positive terminal of the battery loses electrons to the battery.
- ❖ Once it is charged the capacitor has the same voltage as of the battery.
- ❖ Here you have a battery, a light bulb, and a capacitor. If the capacitor is big, what you will notice is that when you connect the battery, the light bulb will light up as current flows from the battery to the capacitor to charge it up. The bulb will get progressively dimmer and finally go out once the capacitor reaches its capacity. If you then remove the battery and replace it with a wire, the current will flow from one plate of the capacitor to the other. The bulb will light initially and then dim as the capacitors discharge until it's completely out.
- ❖ **Uses of capacitors:** Capacitors are used for several purposes.
  - *Timing:* For example, with a 555 timer IC controlling the charging and discharging.
  - *Smoothing:* For example, in a power supply.
  - *Coupling:* For example, between stages of an audio system and to connect a loudspeaker.
  - *Filtering:* For example, in the tone control of an audio system.
  - *Tuning:* For example, in a radio system.
- ❖ **Storing energy:** For example, in a camera flash circuit.

■ TRANSISTORS

Although the vacuum tube made many electromedical apparatus possible, scientific researchers searched for a device to transmit and amplify current that was smaller than a vacuum tube.

Properties

- ❖ Transistors are solid-state semiconductors.
- ❖ They are like triode tubes.
- ❖ They differ from the vacuum tubes in several ways:
  - Require little input.
  - Last indefinitely.
  - Considerable amplification.
  - They are superior to vacuum tubes when space, and power are primary factors.

- They can be powered by a battery instead of a house current and because of their size, the instrument can be miniature. For example, hearing aids.

TRANSDUCERS

In some of the physiologic phenomena measures and records are by nature non-electric for example, sound, heat, or motion. An intermediate instrument is needed in such situations to convert that physical quantity into the equivalent electric quantity and measure accordingly.

Parts and Working

The transducer is an apparatus that converts other forms of energy into electric energy so that they can be measured.

Before explaining the use of the transducer, it is necessary to point out that a purely electronic system, an arrangement of electron vacuum tubes or transistors by itself would be of no use in communications. The system must include apparatus to receive stimuli and emit responses. The stimulus-receiving and response giving devices are input and output transducers **(Fig. 11.5)**.

- **An input transducer** may be a microphone or a photoelectric cell. Since the transducer is an energy-converting device, the microphone converts sound energy into electric energy.
- **The output transducer** is sometimes known as a reproducer because it recreates the stimuli in their original form, but usually on a large scale or in a form more conveniently perceived by the observer.

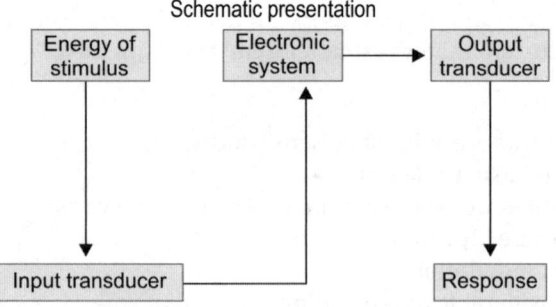

Fig. 11.5: Working of the transducer.

■ COMMON ELECTRIC EQUIPMENT USED IN PATIENT CARE

Thermionic Thermometer

One instrument that changes heat to electric energy is the thermionic thermometer **(Fig. 11.6)**.

Working Principle

Temperature-measuring instrument consists of two wires of different metals joined at each end. One junction is placed where the temperature is to be measured, and the other is kept at a constant lower (reference) temperature. A measuring instrument is connected to the electrical circuit. The temperature difference causes the development of an electromotive force that is approximately proportional to the difference between the temperatures of the two junctions. Temperature can be read from standard tables, or the instrument can be calibrated to display temperature directly **(Fig. 11.7)**.

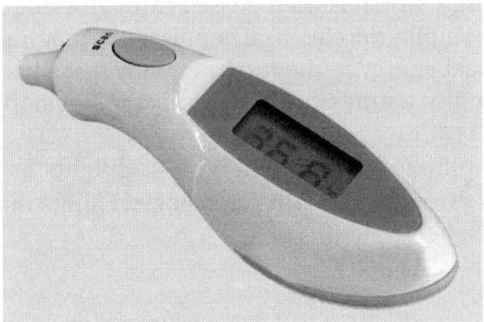

Fig. 11.6: Thermionic thermometer.

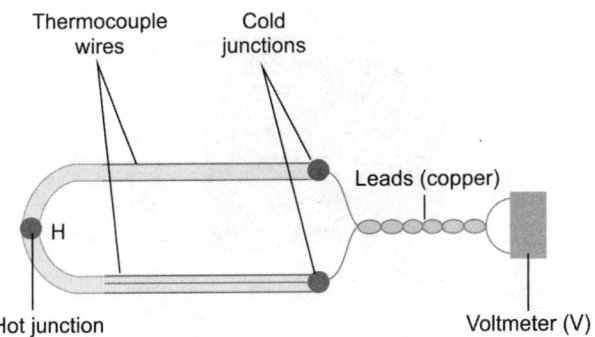

Fig. 11.7: Working of thermionic thermometer.

Uses

- It depends on its action on a crystal that conducts an electric current. The electric resistance of the crystal varies with changes in temperature.
- It is used for obtaining temperatures internally or on the surface of the body.
- The unit is equipped with a variety of probes for obtaining temperatures.
- The thermionic thermometers offer greater accuracy than clinical mercury thermometer can be located up to 1,000 ft from the unit and registers the temperature in about 5 seconds.

Patient Monitors

Patient monitors consist of one or more transducers that are attached to the patient to pick up physiologic information.

Working

As stated, the transducer changes the physiologic information into electrical energy, which is then passed through electronic circuits. These circuits amplify the electrical impulses and may transform them into mechanical energy in the form of a moving stylus that records the patient's pulse temperatures, respiration and blood pressure on a graph **(Fig. 11.8)**.

Other monitors are equipped with flashlights or ring bells if the patient is exceeding certain physiological limits that have been programmed into the circuits.

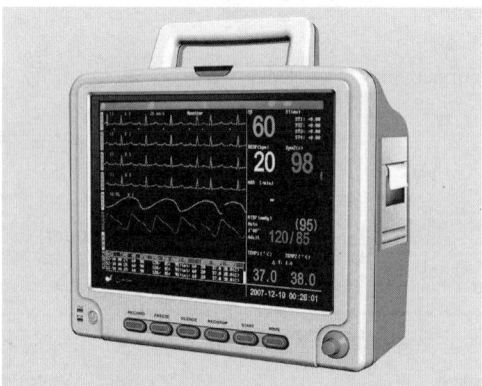

Fig. 11.8: Electronic monitors.

Uses

❖ An apparatus has been reported that during surgery, pick-up impulses from the patient and convert them into lighted numbers on a visible panel where they can be seen readily by a surgeon, nurse, and anesthetist.
❖ Cardioscope, delivers a picture of cardiac activity on a screen in the form of a light flick.
❖ Fetal monitors report the condition of the fetus during pregnancy, labor, and delivery.

Cathode Ray Oscilloscope

It is an important aid to the biophysicist, physiologist, and clinician in the study of the electric potentials in the human body.

Functioning

The basic operation on which the instrument functions is a stream of electrons that are liberated from a hot filament or cathode. The electron stream then passed through an anode at a high potential and strikes a fluorescent screen at the end of the tube. Whenever an electron strike a fluorescent screen a spot of light appears **(Fig. 11.9)**.

Use

The electron stream is deflected from pursuing a straight path by an amplified current, that is received from the part of the body under study. This action current is connected to a pair of horizontal plates that deflect the electrons vertically and vice versa. The picture produced on the screen is a pattern of these deflections as the beam sweeps horizontally across the screen. The light pattern formed may be studied immediately or a photograph may be recorded for future study.

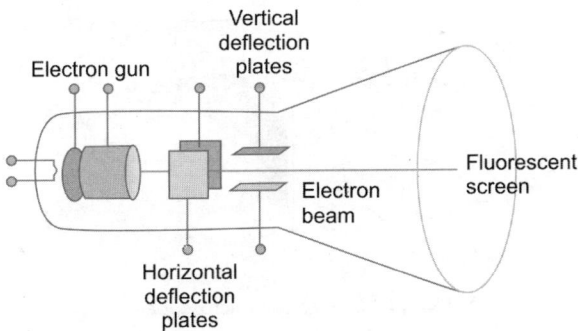

Fig. 11.9: Cathode ray oscilloscope.

Electron Microscope

- It depends upon the properties of the electron for its operation.
- Ordinary microscopes cannot be used to view objects less than 0.000039 cm in diameter which is the same in magnitude as the shortest wavelength of visible light.
- Electrons possess a wave property similar to that of light waves. The wavelength emitted depends upon the voltage with which the electrons are accelerated. Under certain conditions, the wavelength may be 0.05A. This is so much shorter than the shorter wavelength of visible lights (3,900A) that such minute objects as bacteriophage particles have been seen with the aid of the electron microscope.
- The electron beam is provided by an electron gun. It contains an anode with a small opening to allow the electrons to pass through. The anode is grounded while the filament is at a negative voltage of 50,000 or more. There is also a doughnut-shaped coil of wire that acts on electrons like a convex lens, bending them on the object. The electrons beam is altered by the material by being stopped, retarded, or scattered. The electron beam is then passed through another electron lens that corresponds to the objective of the optical microscope. A third lens magnifies the image that is then focused on a fluorescent screen where it may be seen or photographed **(Fig. 11.10)**.

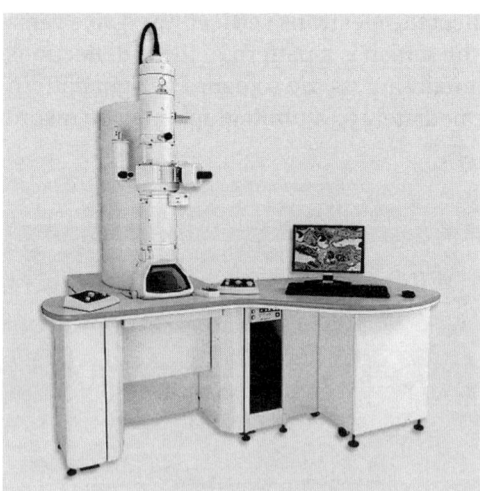

Fig. 11.10: Electron microscope.

- ❖ Difference between electron microscope and ordinary microscope:
  - Stream of fast-moving electrons instead of light rays.
  - Coils of wire in place of lenses.
  - A fluorescent screen or photographic plate instead of an eyepiece.

Diathermy

- ❖ The passage of an electric current through tissues will cause heating. To obtain a significant amount of heat with ordinary low-frequency currents, it would be necessary to use a large amount of current so that the tissue would be destroyed. High-frequency current however may be passed through tissues for a heating effect without causing damage. Diathermy is a means of producing heat in tissues of the body by use of high-frequency electric currents.
- ❖ The heat is generated by induction, which means it is produced without actual contact of the electrodes carrying the current within the tissues.
- ❖ Diathermy uses electromagnetic waves of higher frequencies than infrared radiations

Uses

- ❖ Diathermy has been reported effective in traumatic and inflammatory conditions of the skeleton for relief of bronchitis and pain of pleurisy.
- ❖ Ultra high-frequency diathermy may be used for inducing fever. This reaction known as electro pyrexia is of value in the treatment of general paresis.

Application of Electronics in Nursing

1. **Application in assessment:** Many electronic equipments are used for assessment and routine check-up of health conditions such as digital and thermionic thermometer for temperature, BP monitor for measuring blood pressure and pulse, and auscultation and recording of heart and lung sounds with a digital stethoscope. Assessment of glucose level in blood with glucometer for diabetes and hemoglobin for anemia also level of oxygen in the blood is assessed through oximeter.
   - To assess the heart condition through ECG and mental condition with EEG is possible by electronics.
- ❖ **Application in continuous monitoring:** Monitors are providing continuous data regarding vitals inwards, ICU, and operation rooms to take early necessary action if the condition is about to deteriorate.

Nowadays, smartwatches and mobile technology is providing continuous data related to the health and fitness of a person, this may be used for tracking and monitoring especially to geriatric and specially-abled persons.
- Electronic fetal monitoring measures the response of the fetus's heart rate to contractions of the uterus. It provides an ongoing record. As a nurse, we should be able to read and review the electronic recording of the fetus's heartbeat. A pair of belts are wrapped around the abdomen of mother. One belt uses Doppler to detect the fetal heart rate. The other belt measures the length of contractions and the time between them.

❖ **Application in treatment and follow-up:** Medication dispenser for the elderly people to have in time medication with the correct amount of doses.
- The pacemaker is used to resolve the missing heartbeat or slow heartbeat by generating electrical pulses and bringing the heart back to working condition as a nurse, we should know the normal and abnormal ECG patterns with the pacemaker.
- Neural stimulator relieves the pain signals between the spinal cord and the brain by generates electrical impulses and soothes the body quickly. As a nurse, we should be able to identify malfunction early as miss firing or hyper-firing.
- Triaxial accelerometer and many other sensors are being used to monitor the activity level of patients. Many sensors are being used in physiotherapy to track and correct the exercise patterns so we should know the proper positioning and use of them.
- During surgery, the anesthesia machine is maintained the levels of gases like oxygen, air, nitrous oxide, and isoflurane. For this purpose, sensors are required to control temperature, humidity, and pressure. There is a water lock to prevent seepage of water in a machine that should be monitored regularly and changed periodically, and a nurse should know the functioning basics so malfunctioning is identified early.
- As nursing person, we should know the changing technologies and proper use them, in the near future, we will be surrounded by so many electronic sensors to help us from assessment to implementation and evaluation of care with adequate follow-up and feedbacks.
- Automated IV pumps control the dosages and drips given to patients. Software and medical tech allow nurses to change the drip amounts and medication doses so patients aren't waiting for changes. There are IV pumps for nutrition that give needed

meals at the right times. Additionally, there are self-pumps that allow patients to increase a controlled amount of pain medication for themselves. Automated IV pumps help speed up nursing processes and can be crucial if there is a need for immediate adjustment. Changing medication through an automated process also removes elements of human error that could present issues for clinical patients and hospitals.
- Electronic health records (EHR) are replacing older paper filing methods. Electronic health records allow nursing experts to document care provided to patients and retrieve information that can help prioritize care. Additionally, information entered into computer systems can then be accessed by the care team, including doctors and even patients themselves when necessary.
- Telehealth is a valuable, newer element in healthcare. Hospitals and clinics allow patients to virtually video chat with a doctor or nurse to describe their symptoms or show doctors things like rashes or bumps. This helps patients with a quick diagnosis without leaving the comfort of their own home. They can find out if they need to come in for further testing or diagnosis, get a prescription for medicine, or get medical advice.
- Telehealth saves both patients and doctors money and time. Similarly, it prevents sick patients from coming to public places and exposing other patients. This technology is changing the way clinics operate and how patients are cared for.

■ QUESTIONS

Q.1: Describe about vacuum tubes.
Q.2: Discuss about common electronic equipment used in patient care.

■ BIBLIOGRAPHY

1. Bullock TH. Electroreception, Springer, 2005.
2. Flitter HH, Rowe HR. An Introduction to Physics in Nursing. St Louis: The CV Mosby Company, 1995.
3. Gomber KL, Gogia KL. Fundamental Physics. Ambala: Paedeep Publishers, 2004.
4. Goyal RP, Tripathi SP. Oncise Physics, New Delhi: Selina Publishers, August 2007.
5. Jackson MB. Molecular and Cellular Biophysics. New York: Cambridge Publication, 2006.
6. Lal S. Principles of Physics. Ambala: Paedeep Publishers, 2004.
7. Mielczarek EV, Greenbaum E, Knox RS. Biological Physics. New York. American Institute of Physic, 1993.

8. Morris SC. Life's Solution: Inevitable Humans in a Lonely Universe, Cambridge University Press, 2003.
9. Margaret Scisney-Matlock, Donna Algase, Susan Boehm, Patricia Coleman-Burns, Deborah Oakley, Ann E. Rogers. SeonAe Yeo, Erica Young, and Mei-yu Yu. Measuring Behavior: Electronic Devices in Nursing Studies .Applied Nursing Research, Vol. 13, No. 2 (May), 2000: pp 97–102

Index

Page numbers followed by *f* refer to figure and *t* refer to table.

A

Absolute humidity 73
Absorption 141
Acceleration 17
    average 18
    types of 18
Accidents, inertia in 19
Accommodation, power of 96
Achilles tendon 53
Acne vulgaris 107
Agricultural research 213
Air pressure 113
Alcohol 22
Alpha-radiation 207
Alpha-waves 180
Aluminum 22
Amniotic sac 120
Amplitude 138, 138*f*
Analog circuits 224
Angina 182
Antiseptics, surface tension of 4
Aphakia 97
Applanation method 128
Aqueous humor 114
Archimedes' principle 28*f*
    applications of 28
Arterial blood pressure 114
Arterial pressure 125
    measuring 126
Arthritis, diagnosis of 107
Artificial radiation sources 209
Astigmatism 97, 100
Atmospheric pressure 115
    applications of 117
Atom
    Bohr's model of 200
    orbits of 200*f*, 203*f*
    structure of 197
Atomic physics 5
Audiogram 155
Audiometers 147
Audiometry 4, 147
Auditory neuropathy spectrum disorder 154
Autoclave 4
Automated external defibrillators 189, 189*f*, 191

B

Bactericidal effects 107
Bad and semiconductor 162*f*

Balanced traction 60, 60*f*
Balmer series 204
Basal metabolic rate 48
Basal metabolism 4
Basic life support 189
Battery force 167
Becker bolt 129
Beta-radiation 208
Beta-waves 180
Biological methods 124
Biophysics 1, 2
    importance of 2
Birds respirator oxygen tent 117
Bismuth-213 211
Blood
    circulation of 4
    plasma 22
    viscosity of 4
Body
    alignment 31
    balance 31
    mechanics 50
        principles of 51
    part of 219
    pressure 114
    radiation effects on 215
    temperature, regulation of 77
Bohr's model 204
Bohr's theory 204
Boiling point 72
Boyle's law 122
Brackett series 203, 204
Brain
    pacemaker 186, 187*f*
    pressure in 114
Breathing 121
British thermal unit 66
Buoyant force 27*f*
Burger's capillary glass tube method 125

C

Calorie 45
    value 48
Capacitor 227, 228*f*
    diagrammatic presentation of 228*f*
    uses of 229
Capillary blood pressure 114
Carbohydrate 48
Cardiac pacemakers 4
Cardiovascular disease 59
Cat scan 193
Cathode ray oscilloscope 233, 233*f*

Celsius and Fahrenheit scale 75f, 76
Centigrade scale 75
Centimeter-gram-second system 6, 7
Central venous pressure 126
    measuring 126
Centrifugal force 41, 42, 43f
Centrifuge devices, motion in 18
Cerebrospinal fluid 114, 129
Cervical traction 58
Cesium-131 211
Charged body, discharging of 163
Charges, flow of 166f
Charles's law 122
Chemical effects 172
Chest 188, 194
Chromium-51 211
Circadian rhythm 103
Circular motion 16
    forces in 41
Claustrophobia 59
Clinical thermometer 76
Cobalt-57 212
Cold application, application of 4
Colloidal dispersions 4
Combustion, heat of 73
Common electric equipment 231
Communication system, picture exchange 154
Compression 135
Computed axial tomography 193
Computed tomography 191, 193
Concave lens 94f, 99f
Condensation, heat of 73
Conduction 68, 161
Conductive hearing loss 153
Conductors, applications of 69
Constructive interference 142f
Convection 69
Convex lens 98f
    case of 93f
Copper-64 212
Corpuscle's theory of light, failures of 85
Coulomb's law 161, 175
Current 166
Curvature hyperopia 97

D

Dalton's law 122
Davis social adequacy index 148
Defibrillation 187, 188f
Delta-waves 180
Derived units 5
Destructive interference 142f
Device 168
Diagnostic reference level 217
Diathermy 4, 150f, 235
Digital circuits 225
Diode 225
    tube 225, 226f

Direct ionizing radiation 207
Discrimination score 148
Distant vision, least distance of 96
Domain theory 177, 178f
Doppler effect 145
Dosimeters 221
Dynamic 16
    contour tonometry 128

E

Echocardiography 151
Echoencephalography 151
Education 156
Elastic waves 134
Elasticity 133
Electric 158
    cautery 172f
    current 166
        chemical source of 169
        effects of 171
    motors 173f
    shock therapy 4
Electricity 4, 158
    magnetic sources of 170
    mechanical sources of 170
    phenomenon of 158
    radiant source of 168
    thermal source of 169
    types of 159
Electrification, theory of 160, 160f
Electrocardiogram 182f
Electrocardiography 181
Electroconvulsive therapy 184
    machine 185f
Electrodynamics 159, 166
Electroencephalogram 180f
Electroencephalography 179
Electromagnet 173
Electromagnetic waves 134
Electromagnetism 158
Electromotive force 167
Electromyography 183, 183f
    pattern 183
Electron
    beam tomography 194
    microscope 234, 234f
Electronic 224
    application of 235
    cardiac pacemaker 185
    circuit with resistance 167f
    devices 130
    health records 237
    monitors 232f
    principles of 225
Electrostatic 159
    applications of 164
    precipitation 164, 165f
Electrostimulation 184
Electrosurgical procedures 4

Index

Endocrines 102
Energy 45
    conservation of 48
    conversion factor 46t
    in body 47
    level 188
    transformation of 46
    types of 46
English systems 11t
Environment preparation, use in 80
Environmental protection agency 218
Ergosterol, activation of 107
Erythema, production of 107
Erythrocyte sedimentation 28
Evaporation 70
Exfoliation 107
Exposed persons, protection of 156
External cardiac pacemaker 186f
Eye
    action of 95
    pressure 114
    structure of 95, 95f

■ F

Fahrenheit scale 75
Far sightedness 97, 99
Fats 48
Fetal heart monitoring 151
Field strength 176
Film badge dosimeter 221
First class lever 51, 52f
Fluid
    flows 121
    mechanics 113
    movement 30
    volume 9
Fluorine 212
Focal length 93
Food 48
    preservation and sterilization 214
    types 48t
Foot
    lever action of 53, 54f
    pound-second system 6, 7
Force 3, 34
    energy and work 34
Forearm, lever action of 54, 55f
Freezing points 71, 71f
Frequency 138
Friction, principles of 40
Frictional force 39
Fundamental units 5, 6
Fusion, heat of 72

■ G

Gallium 212
Gamma radiation 208
Gastrointestinal pressure 114
Geiger-Muller counter 204
Generators, working of 171f
Glucose 48
Gold 22
Goldmann tonometry 128
Good conductors 162f
Gravitational force 41
    effects of 28
Gravity 3, 21, 32
    application of principles of 28, 62
    edema due to 31f
    force of 35
    IV fluid administration with 30f
    principles of 26, 28, 29
    specific 3, 22, 22t
    center of 3, 23, 23f, 24f
Guinea pigs 102

■ H

Hamburger's red corpuscle method 124
Health aspects 103
Healthcare practices 65
Hearing 144
    aids 146
    assistive technology system 154
    loss 153
        interpreting 148t
        mixed 154
Heart 4
Heat 4, 65, 66, 82
    application, application of 4
    measurement of 66
    nature of 65
    on matter, effects of 71
    principles, application of 79
    quantitative measure of 66
    specific 74
    transfer of 68
    transmission 71f
High energy radiation 5
Hill's method 125
Hip joint 54
Human audibility 4
Human beings, mechanical efficiency of 50t
Human body 28
    effects of electricity on 173
Human health effects 152
Humidity 73
    specific 74
Hydraulic brakes 120
Hydraulic carjacks 120
Hydrogen, spectrum of 202f
Hydrostatic pressure 119
Hypermetropia 97, 98f
Hyperopia 97
    axial 97
    simple 97
Hyperthermia 80, 81

I

Index hyperopia 97
Indium 212
Induction 162
　　process of 162
Industrial use 214
Infection 59
Infrared radiation 105
Instantaneous acceleration 18
Instantaneous velocity 17
Intensity 140, 143
Intensive care units 224
Interference 141
International system of units 6, 66
Intra-abdominal pressure 129
Intracranial pressure 129
　　measuring 129
Intraocular pressure 114, 127, 128
　　measuring 128
Invasive methods 129
Iodine 212
Ionizing radiation 207, 221
　　detection of 221
Iron 22, 212
Irregular reflection 91
Isotopes 206

J

Jaw, lever action of 53, 53f
Joint problems 59

K

Kelvin scales 76
Kidney, artificial 4
Kilogram calorie 45
Kilowatt-hour 46
Kinematics 16
Kinetic energy 47f, 125, 133

L

Ladd device 130
Ladd fiber optic system 129
Lead 22, 212
Legislation 156
Length, units of 6, 7t
Lens 92, 93
　　absence of 97
　　actions of 4
　　basic features of 93f
　　features of 93
Lethal 150
Lever 51
　　representation 55f, 56f
Light 84
　　application of principles of 110
　　biological effects of 100
　　corpuscular theory of 85
　　diffuse and smooth reflection of 90f
　　energy 84
　　nature of 84
　　quantum theory of 86
　　reflection of 89, 89f, 90f
　　refraction of 88, 89f, 91, 92, 92f
　　uses of 104
　　wave theory of 85, 86
Lightening rod 163f
Liver action 54, 56
Locomotion, effect on 100
Longitudinal wave motion 135, 136f
Long-sightedness 97
Lumbar puncture 120, 130
Lyman series 204

M

Machine
　　mechanical advantage of 50
　　principles of 49
　　simple 49
Magnet, applications of 178
Magnetic attraction 175f
Magnetic devices 179f
Magnetic fields 175
Magnetic force, law of 175
Magnetic inductions 176
Magnetic lines of force, characteristics of 176
Magnetic moment 177
Magnetic repulsion 176f
Magnetic resonance imaging 16, 191, 192f
　　nuclear 191
Magnetism 174
　　applications of 178
Manmade radiation 211
Manometer 124, 127
Mass 24, 26
　　and weight, unit of 8
Measurement 3
　　units of 35
Mechanical effects 172
Mechanical methods 123
Mechanical wave 134, 136
Medicine, visible light in 105
Melting points 71, 71f
Mercury 22
　　advantages of 68
　　thermometer, construction of 68
Metabolism
　　effect on 100
　　tracer studies of 5
Metre-kilogram-second system 6, 7
Metric system 7, 8, 11t
Microscopy 4
Middle ear pressure 114
Mirrors, use of 4
Molecular physics 4
Motion 3, 13, 19

Index

applications of 18
during walking 18
sickness 18
third law of 38
types of 15
Movable pulleys 57
Multi-element tube 226
Muscle action 3
Musical sound 142
Myopia 97, 98
    corrected 99f

N

Natural radiation sources 209
Neutron radiation 208
Newton's first law 36
Newton's law of motion 35
Newton's second law 37
Newton's third law 38
Newton's universal law 41
Newton's words 38
Noise 143, 152
    pollution 152
        prevention of 155
    sources of 152
Noninvasive methods 129
Nonionizing radiation 209
Nuclear physics 197
Nuclear regulatory commission 218

O

Ocular pathologic conditions 97
Ohm's law 168
Operation
    mechanism of 190
    theatres 224
Ophthalmoscope 4
Optic axis 93
Optical center 93
Oral thermometer 77f
Organ pressure 114
Orifice, area of 121
Orthostatic hypotension 19
Oscillatory motion 16
Osmotic pressure 122, 123
    applications of 125
    measurement of 123, 123f
Osteoporosis 59

P

P wave 181
Paddle placement 188
Paddle size 188
Paddle-skin interface material 188
Pain 81
Palladium 212
Pascal's law 119
    applications of 119

principle of 120
    working applications of 120f
Paschen series 203, 204
Patient care 231
Patient handling 32
Patient monitors 232
Pentode tube 226
Pfund series 203, 204
Phonocardiography 182
Photoelectric
    cell 169f
    effect 86f
Photokinesis 100
Photomultiplier tube 222
Photoperiodicity 101
Photoperiodism 101
Photosensitivity 101, 110, 111f
    reactions 110
Physical methods 124
Pigmentation effects 101
Pinnotheres maculatus 100
Pitch 143
Platinum 22
Pneumatonometry 128
Polarity 174
Positional hyperopia 97
Positron emission tomography 213
Potassium-42 212
Potential energy 47f, 133
Power 49
Pregnancy 59
Presbyopia 97, 99
Pressure 4, 113, 114
    gradient 121
    importance of 114
    measurement of 125
    typical value of 114, 114t
    wave 135
Principal axis 93
Principal focus 93
Proportional counting chamber 205
Protective coloration 101
Proteins 48
Psoriasis 107
Pulley 57, 57f
Pulse formation 4
Pure water 22
Purkinje fibers 182

Q

QRS complex 182
Quantum, light in form of 87f
Quartz fiber dosimeter 221

R

Radiant effects 171
Radiation 70, 107, 206
    artificial 211
    classification 207

indirect ionizing 208
internal sources of 210
protection
basic three factors for 220
limits 218
Radioactive material, use of 5
Radioactive substances, naturally occurring 206
Radioactivity and monitoring, detection of 204
Radiofrequency 191
Radioisotope 5, 206, 211, 212
applications 211
exposure effects 215
Radiological protection 220
Radiotherapy, half-life in 5
Radiotracer 211
Radium-223 212
Rapid eye movement 103
Rarefaction 136
Ray
reflection of 140f
refraction of 141f
Red blood cell, fate of 124f
Red cells 124
Reflection 140
law of 88
regular 90
types of 90
uses of 91
Refraction 4, 91, 141
Refractive index 91
Relative humidity 73
importance of 74
Resistance 167
Rest and motion 15
Rhenium-186 212
Rheumatoid arthritis 59
Richmond screw 129
Rotational motion 16
Rubidium-82 212
Russell traction 60, 61f
Rutherford's model of atom 198
Rutherford's scattering experiment 199f

■ S

Scalar and vector quantity 14f
Scalar quantity 13, 14t
Scalars and vectors 13
Scintillation counters 205, 222
Screw 62
Second class lever 52, 52f
Sedation 180
Sensorineural hearing loss 153
Shadow, casting of 88f
Shielding 218
Shock, frequency of 188
Short sightedness 97, 98
SI system 7

Siphon 118, 118f
Skeletal muscles 4
Skeletal traction 58
Skin traction 58
Snell's law 91
Sodium chloride solution 122
Sodium-24 212
Solidification, heat of 72
Sonar navigation 149f
and ranging 149
Sound
characteristics of 142
waves 132, 137
Speech
audiometry 148
reception threshold 148
Speed 16
Spinal fluid flow test 120
Static electricity 159, 159f
Steam inhalation 4
Sterile insect technique 214
Sterilization 4
use of heat for 79
Stethoscope 146, 146f
Storing energy 229
ST-segment 182
Sublimation 73
Symbalophone 147

■ T

T wave 182
Telehealth 237
Temperature 66
on magnet, effect of 177
scales 75
Terrestrial radiation sources 209
Thallium-201 212
Thermal capacity 75t
Thermal effects 171
Thermal energy 66, 78t
Thermionic thermometer 231, 231f
working of 231f
Thermocouple 169f
Thermography 4, 106, 106f
Thermoluminescent dosimeter 221
Thermometer 67f
Thermometric substance 68
Thermometry 4
Third class lever 52, 52f
Thomas splint traction 60f
Thomson's atomic model 197, 198f
Thomson's model 198
Thorium protactinium beta particle 208
Three-dimensional volumetric information 195
Time, units of 10
Tonometry 128
Torricelli experiment 115f
Torricellian vacuum 115

Index

Traction, purpose of 57
Transcranial Doppler 129
Transducer 127, 230
  output 230
  working of 230f
Transistors 229
  use of 4
Translatory motion 15
Transmission 141
Transverse wave motion 134, 135f
Triode tube 226, 227f
Tumor, diagnosis of 107
Tuning forks 155
Tympanic membrane displacement 129
Typical energy values 48t

U

U wave 182
Ultrasonic sound waves 149
  adverse effects of 150
  production of 150
Ultrasonic wave 149
Ultrasound 151
  diathermy 150
  uses of 150
Ultraviolet radiation 107
Uniform circular motion 41
Uniform velocity 17
Unit 109
  concept of 5
  systems of 6, 7t
Uranium
  fuel cycle 220
  thorium alpha particle 208
Urinary bladder 114

V

Vacuum tubes 225
  types of 225
Vapor
  pressure 72, 72f
  tension, noting 125
Vaporization, heat of 73
Variable velocity 17
Vector 14t
  quantities 14
Vehicles, control of 156
Velocity 16, 139
  average 17
  types of 17

Venous and arterial systems 129
Venous blood pressure 114
Ventilation phase 188
Ventricular dysrhythmias 187
Ventricular fibrillation 187
Ventricular tachycardia 187
Visible light, application of 105f
Vision
  defects of 97
  physics of 94
Visual fields 4
Vitamin D 107
Vocalization 144
Voltaic cell 170f

W

Water, exercise in and out of 29f
Waves
  mechanism of propagation of 133, 133f
  non-mechanical 134
  pattern 181
  phenomenon 140
Wave motion 133, 138
  types of 134
Wavelength 139, 139f
Weaknesses 204
Weight 9, 24, 26
  and measurements, conversion of 9t
Whole blood 22
Wolff-Parkinson-White syndrome 182
Work 44
  and energy 4
  measurement of 44

X

X-ray 108, 109, 221
  radiation 208
  therapy 5

Y

Ytterbium-169 212

Z

Zinc sulfate 198